MEDICAL
INTELLIGENCE
UNIT

NOVEL CHEMOTHERAPEUTIC AGENTS: PREACTIVATION IN THE TREATMENT OF CANCER AND AIDS

Kirpal S. Gulliya, Ph.D.

Director of Immunophotobiology and Drug Development
Baylor University Medical Center
Baylor Research Institute
Dallas, Texas, U.S.A.

Associate Professor, Institute of Biomedical Studies
Baylor University
Waco, Texas, U.S.A.

Professor (adjunct), Department of Biological Sciences
University of North Texas
Denton, Texas, U.S.A.

Springer-Verlag Berlin Heidelberg GmbH

MEDICAL INTELLIGENCE UNIT

NOVEL CHEMOTHERAPEUTIC AGENTS:
PREACTIVATION IN THE TREATMENT OF CANCER AND AIDS

R.G. LANDES COMPANY
Austin, Texas, U.S.A.

Springer

International ISBN 978-3-662-22243-0

While the authors, editors and publisher believe that drug selection and dosage and the specifications and usage of equipment and devices, as set forth in this book, are in accord with current recommendations and practice at the time of publication, they make no warranty, expressed or implied, with respect to material described in this book. In view of the ongoing research, equipment development, changes in governmental regulations and the rapid accumulation of information relating to the biomedical sciences, the reader is urged to carefully review and evaluate the information provided herein.

Library of Congress Cataloging-in-Publication Data

Gulliya, K.S. (Kirpal S.)
Novel chemotherapeutic agents : preactivation in the treatment of cancer and AIDS / K.S. Gulliya
p. cm. — (Medical intelligence unit)
Includes bibliographical references and index.
ISBN 978-3-662-22243-0 ISBN 978-3-662-22241-6 (eBook)
DOI 10.1007/978-3-662-22241-6
1.Cancer—Photochemotherapy. 2.AIDS (Disease)—Photochemotherapy. I. Title. II.Series.
[DNLM: 1. Neoplasms—drug therapy. 2. Acquired Immunodeficiency Syndrome—drug therapy. 3. Antineoplastic Agents. 4. Antiviral Agents. 5. Photosensitizing Agents. 6. Chemistry, Pharmaceutical—United States. QZ 267 G973n 1996]
RC271.P43G85 1996 616.99'4061—dc20
DNLM/DLC 96-17729
for Library of Congress CIP

Publisher's Note

R.G. Landes Company publishes six book series: *Medical Intelligence Unit, Molecular Biology Intelligence Unit, Neuroscience Intelligence Unit, Tissue Engineering Intelligence Unit, Biotechnology Intelligence Unit* and *Environmental Intelligence Unit.* The authors of our books are acknowledged leaders in their fields and the topics are unique. Almost without exception, no other similar books exist on these topics.

Our goal is to publish books in important and rapidly changing areas of bioscience and environment for sophisticated researchers and clinicians. To achieve this goal, we have accelerated our publishing program to conform to the fast pace in which information grows in bioscience. Most of our books are published within 90 to 120 days of receipt of the manuscript. We would like to thank our readers for their continuing interest and welcome any comments or suggestions they may have for future books.

Deborah Muir Molsberry
Publications Director
R.G. Landes Company

Dedication

This book is dedicated to cancer and AIDS patients and their families throughout the world and to my family, parents and brother, Om Parkash.

CONTRIBUTING AUTHOR

Anthony A. Harriman, Ph.D.
Professor, Laboratoire de Photochimie
Ecole Europeénne Chimie Polymeres Materiaux
Université Louis Pasteur
Strasbourg Cedex, France

AUTHOR'S NOTE

Regarding Dr. Harriman's contribution to the subject of preactivation, it must also be noted that the manner in which he stood steadfast took courage, integrity, and insight to pursue this project (which was only of ancillary interest to him), for the sake of knowledge and science. His decision to stay the course, fully aware of the professional risks in association with a novel idea in its infancy, speaks volumes about the character of the man. I do not have sufficient words to express my gratitude to have had the opportunity to work with a true scientist.

K.S. Gulliya

CONTENTS

PREFACE

This book describes the discovery of a new technology termed "preactivation." Preactivation is a process by which photoactive compounds are first exposed to light and thereby converted into new potential drugs that function independent of light. Basic and preclinical studies have revealed the dramatic therapeutic potential of some of these compounds. Thus, preactivation can be used to convert thousands of existing photoactive compounds into new potential anticancer and antiviral agents.

Although the process of preactivation uses a principle of photodynamic therapy, the resulting products are strictly chemotherapeutic in nature, in that they function independent of light. Once identified, the photoproducts generated via the process of preactivation can be chemically synthesized.

Therapeutic use of light energy by itself or as an activating agent for light-reactive chemicals dates back to ancient Egypt. Since those times, one fundamental principle of photodynamic therapy has remained constant: light energy is always applied after the light-reactive chemical or photoactive agent has arrived at the target. The basis for this rationale is that the singlet oxygen generated upon illumination, thought to be the sole cause of tumor damage, has a very short half-life (micro- or milliseconds). Also, controlling the area of illumination limits collateral damage to the adjacent tissue. However, for the target (e.g. tumor) to be illuminated it has to be large enough to be visible to the naked eye and accessible to light via fiber optics or surgery.

Since light cannot penetrate the human body, a major drawback of this approach is that photodynamic therapy cannot be used for the treatment of systemic diseases or viral infections because the tumor cell itself or the virus is too small to be visible to the naked eye, and thus, practically speaking, cannot be selectively illuminated. Indeed, because of this major limitation of photodynamic therapy, it has been stated that "the dependence on light to deliver the coup de grâce may one day be viewed as barbarically primitive."[†]

That day has been here for at least the past nine years. This book describes how the process of preactivation generates novel compounds that exert their tumor cell preferential cytotoxicity independent of light and thus, unlike photodynamic therapy, can be used for systemic therapy of malignancies, metastases and viral infections. Compounds thus generated are stable for long periods of time and can be stored for later use.

Experiments with preactivation also show that the prevailing thinking, which maintains that singlet oxygen produced at excited states is the sole

---

[†] *Clinical Oncology Alert, December 1993; 8:89-96.*

destroyer of tumor cells in photodynamic therapy, is wrong. This conclusion is based on the following observations:

1.) The role of singlet oxygen generated at excited states as a sole destroyer of tumor cells has never been proven.
2.) There is no correlation between the yield of singlet oxygen and the quantity of tumor cell kill. A case in point is the compound merocyanine 540 which is a very poor producer of singlet oxygen yet very effective in killing tumor cells upon appropriate illumination. This tumor cell destruction is at least as good or better than the one obtained by the use of a hematoporphyrin derivative, which is an excellent producer of singlet oxygen.
3.) Even if one assumes that singlet oxygen is the sole destroyer of tumor cells, dark toxicity of preactivated compounds cannot be explained because the half-life and diffusion range of singlet oxygen in aqueous media are extremely short.
4.) At least for one photoactive compound, merocyanine 540, experiments have demonstrated that the role of singlet oxygen generated at excited states is more towards attacking the photoactive compound itself and generating new cytotoxic compounds rather than reacting with the target.

In subsequent chapters, the discovery of the preactivation technology as well as the biological effects of novel compounds derived from the process are described. The first chapter addresses serious problems that prevent the development of effective yet easily tolerated drugs because they do not meet the current criteria of drug selection. The challenges and simple corrective measures delineated would open up new opportunities in drug development. The second chapter presents a history of events that led to the discovery and development of chemotherapeutic compounds generated by the application of the novel process of preactivation. The third chapter describes the photochemistry and photophysics of the lead compound used in the process and provides experimental proof of the mechanism(s) involved in the generation of new compounds. In the fourth chapter observations made during the in vitro studies are tested in animal models to demonstrate that these compounds indeed are effective against solid tumors as well as viral infections including HIV-1, and do not produce observable side effects at therapeutic doses. In the fifth chapter, the role of topoisomerases, apoptosis and the involvement of mitochondria as an intracellular target, in the mechanism of action of novel preactivated compounds is described. The concluding chapter presents a brief description of the molecular basis of carcinogenesis and the recently discovered effects of a preactivated compound on the modulation of oncogenes in leukemia.

K.S.G.

Acknowledgments

I am indebted to many people for their interest, support and research collaborations during the course of the development of preactivation technology leading to many co-authored publications and patents. I also want to thank Dr. John Nemunitis, Dr. Daniel Von Hoff and the staff of the Human Tumor Cloning Laboratory for their invaluable collaboration.

I am deeply indebted to Dr. Charles R. Smart, then Chief of Early Detection Branch at NCI for his encouragement to pursue this discovery which he characterized as "a breakthrough" in the field. His comments have been a driving force for me to continue to develop this technology. My special thanks to Dr. R. K. Sharma for reviewing chapter 6 and portions of chapter 5 and for long hours and many weekends he spent in the laboratory conducting experiments; Dr. Shazib Pervaiz of my laboratory for performing many initial experiments on this project; Dr. Frank Bernal-Sogandares for his assistance with in vivo experiments and the staff of our Scientific Publication Office, in particular Ms. Beverly Peters, for rapid preparation of several graphs for this book.

Above all, I am most grateful to Dr. James L. Matthews, Dr. Anthony Harriman, Dr. Buchard Franck, Mr. Sidney Levit and the Leukemia Association of North Central Texas for their undying support even in the face of politics and associated potential repercussions. Clearly without the support of these individuals as well as those appearing on various publications and patents, the progress made in firmly establishing this technology would have been a significantly more difficult task. It is impossible to acknowledge properly here many co-workers who carried out most of the work presented in this book. I have included some names where the opportunity presented itself. However in no case could I do proper justice to everyone's essential roles. I hope they will understand.

I am also grateful to the staff of R. G. Landes Company, in particular Ms. Deborah Molsberry, Ms. Lynn O'Neill, Ms. Valerie Uzcátegui and Dr. Renate Wise. Dr. Landes' invitation to write this book, followed by ebullience, efficiency, support and understanding of the staff members helped to make this undertaking a pleasant experience.

CHAPTER 1

CHALLENGES AND OPPORTUNITIES IN NEW DRUG DEVELOPMENT

Progress in medical science depends chiefly on the uncommon man, possessed of that rare asset, a brain so beautifully integrated with the retina, that when he looks, he perceives. —David Seegal, Journal of Medical Education 1964; 39:321.

In the 18th century, mercury was the treatment of choice for syphilis.[1] Mercury was so commonly used, in fact, that physicians rarely saw a patient who had not taken it, even though it was eventually proven ineffective.[2] As a result, it was virtually impossible to separate the effects of the disease from the treatment. Many physicians even insisted that mercury had no toxic effects.

We are in a similar situation today with cancer treatment. We treat patients with bluntly toxic materials possessing a narrow window of safety, insuring that along with any therapeutic effects the patient will also experience toxic side effects.[3-5] So ingrained are these toxic effects in the public's mind that many patients today associate cancer with wasting, hair loss, infection, vomiting and bleeding, not realizing that these are side effects of the drugs used to treat cancer rather than the symptoms of cancer itself.

Although notable progress has been made in limiting the toxicities of cancer drugs, when we study cancer treatment, we are essentially studying the human responses to toxic agents. Anticancer

Novel Chemotherapeutic Agents: Preactivation in the Treatment of Cancer and AIDS, by K. S. Gulliya.

drugs are powerful toxic agents with an extremely narrow therapeutic index. In most cases the biologically inactive doses may be within one log of lethal dose.[6] In effect, cancer treatment is a huge experiment in the use of toxic substances on human patients.

An observer might point out that there are chilling similarities between this situation and the experiments in which the government secretly exposed human subjects to radiation during World War II, leaving them vulnerable to wasting, leukemia and other delayed effects. How, in fact, are the two cases different? The answer is that cancer patients are told beforehand the agent to be used, the potential therapeutic effect and the potential for toxic side effects.

The typical pre-treatment explanation of potential toxic effects simply does not convey what the experience of the effects will be like, however. The ordeal of cancer treatment itself has led some patients to state that if they had even a remote idea of the difficulties, discomfort and agonies that chemotherapy may bring, they would have preferred to die untreated.

The profound intensity of these kinds of statements, obviously arising from intense suffering, is reason enough to launch an all-out effort in search of easily tolerated therapeutic compounds. But do such drugs even exist? If so, why has no one found them? The answer is, "yes," they do exist. Why they have not been discovered is a key point of which some of the elements are described below.

How does one find these easily tolerated drugs that also kill cancer? One approach that answers this question is addressed in this book. In the subsequent chapters, it will be demonstrated that it is entirely possible to find drugs that are not only effective against malignancies and viral infections, but that are also easily tolerated. Achievement of this mission has required taking an entirely different approach to drug development, one believed by some to be impossible. This discovery shows that to get different results, one must take a different—or at least less trodden—path. However, to do so, one must give up some currently established paradigms.

A word of caution is in order for those who wish to embark on such an endeavor. Anyone seeking a different path must be prepared for the wrath of friends, colleagues and funding agencies accustomed to doing business based on established paradigms. Self- (or otherwise) proclaimed gurus of the scientific community will be liberal in the kind of illogical criticism one may not have thought possible from learned people who were supposed to have devoted their lives to the search for truth and the betterment of mankind.

Returning back to the central question as to why easily tolerated drugs have not been found, it is important to look at the current criteria of drug selection. Therefore, a brief description of the history of drug development and the problems encountered is followed by an analysis of current criteria used to select new drug candidates for further research and development.

The first major broadly based, anticancer drug development programs originated at the Sloan-Kettering Institute in the United States, the Chester Beatty Institute in England and the University of Tokyo in Japan. Since 1955, the National Cancer Institute (NCI) also has supported an extensive program to discover and develop new drugs for the treatment of cancer.[7] Now there is increasing cooperation between virtually all major organizations of the world for research on treatment of cancer and development of anticancer drugs.

Notwithstanding some notable progress, a large majority of the scientific and clinical community are dissatisfied with the overall progress in the arena of anticancer drug development. Many of the reasons for this growing dissatisfaction were pointed out in a report in 1987 in which Marsoni et al[8] evaluated the Phase II activity of all cytotoxic drugs the National Cancer Institute introduced into trial between 1970 and 1985. Eighty-three drugs were introduced, out of which five drugs remained in Phase I trials. Eleven others were eliminated. Of the 67 drugs progressing to Phase II trials, 13 were still in these trials and 7 had not been evaluated at the time the report was issued. The remaining 47 drugs were considered evaluable for clinical activity, out of which 24 were ranked active against at least one type of cancer.

Since approximately 30% of the drugs identified in preclinical screens turned out to show clinical activity, the data, on the surface, may appear promising. However, Marsoni et al noted several disturbing features in this study. The first major concern was that of the 24 active drugs, only 11 were novel compounds; the other 13 were analogs of known active compounds.

The next serious concern was that 74% of the compounds were found to be active against lymphoma and 35% against leukemia, with only marginal activity against solid tumors. This deficiency was emphasized by Muggia[9] in an accompanying editorial stating that "the criteria for identifying new drugs for clinical development of the National Cancer Institute screens from 1970 to 1985 are unsatisfactory for the detection of clinically useful drugs against these common human cancers." Many inadequacies in the past approaches to cancer drug development were recently described by Grindey.[10]

Since then, the National Cancer Institute has introduced three in vitro test systems to be used as large-scale, primary screens for the selection of new anticancer agents for further research and development. The *first* system is a human tumor colony forming assay originally reported by Hamburger and Salmon.[11] This assay is based on cloning of fresh human tumor cells in primary cultures (semi-solid growth medium) for drug sensitivity testing. Later, it was demonstrated that the susceptibility of a patient's tumor in this assay predicted that the chance of a patient responding clinically to the drug was 81%, while in case of the tumors found to be resistant to the test drug, it predicted that the chance of its clinical failure was 93%.[12]

In subsequent retrospective correlation studies involving 800 patients, Von Hoff et al[13] determined that the true positive and negative rates for this assay were 70% and 80%, respectively. In a more recent prospective clinical trial of the cloning system involving 604 patients, the percent true positive and negative rates for the assay were reported to be 64% and 86%, respectively.[14] Thus, it is clear from these studies that in vitro screening assays can be used for drug screening. However, due to limited availability and access to fresh tumors, this assay cannot be carried out on a large scale.

The National Cancer Institute has instituted a *second* system for in vitro drug screening.[15,16] In this project, new compounds are tested in a panel of more than 60 cell lines derived from seven cancer types. These cell lines have reproducible profiles for growth and drug sensitivity.[17] A protein-binding sulforhodamine dye assay is used to assess cell survival in a dose-response fashion in microtiter plates.[18-21] Tests of known anticancer agents in the screen are used to confirm the pattern of activity in clinical use. (It is very important to note here that new agents are being compared against highly toxic agents that are known for their very narrow therapeutic window.) Even so, it is expected that in addition to identifying new drugs, this new screen will provide the opportunity to pursue disease-oriented screening. Although this program has already identified a few potential compounds, the ability of the screening system to identify new active compounds that eventually prove useful in the clinic remains uncertain.[22,23]

The *third* test system, developed at Wayne State University, is a two tumor disk-diffusion soft agar assay. This assay distinguishes preferential cytotoxicity for the solid tumor cell type over the leukemic cell type. In this system two different tumors, e.g. leukemia (L1210) and a solid (drug insensitive) tumor are co-cultivated on a soft agar disk. The solid tumor cells have the potential for indicating activities of undiscovered, possibly solid tumor-specific antitumor agents. After co-cultivating the two tumor cell lines, the test agent is placed on a filter paper disk on top of the soft agar. At the end of the incubation period with the test drug, cytotoxicity to two different cell lines is evaluated.

However, in order to qualify for further research and development, the new compound must meet the selection criteria developed by the National Cancer Institute. A discussion of these criteria follows.

PRIMARY CRITERIA FOR THE SELECTION OF NEW AGENTS—A CATCH 22

There are five primary criteria for selecting new agents for further research and development. The first requires that the new agent display a pattern of selective toxicity against a specific class of human tumors in the cell line screening assays. The rationale for selecting drugs effective against a specific class of tumors was apparently derived from the expectation that broadly cytotoxic agents would likely cause significant toxicity to normal tissues and would lack specificity for malignant cells, as is the case with our current drugs. If this is indeed the case, then the criterion appears to have been written backwards and this is the major problem in the development of new drugs.

Why not have the first criterion require the new agent to be selectively sparing of normal cells and tissues, while it destroys malignant cells? After all, this is the main goal of cancer therapy, is it not? In its current form, the first criterion appears to have been written to include bluntly toxic agents, because at present there are no anticancer drugs that selectively spare normal cells. In addition, the National Cancer Institute's criterion as written appears to have transformed into an unspoken rule or tradition stating that if the new compound is effective against more than one tumor type, it is no good. This is the main reason new effective anticancer agents that spare the host have never been given a chance to see the light of the day, since they happen to be effective against more than one type of cancer. If there were indeed an agent that spared normal cells and tissues but was toxic to more than one type of tumor, it would be irrelevant whether the drug was specific for tumor type!

In its present form, the first criterion has probably done more to stifle the discovery and development of new easily tolerated drugs than all other factors combined. A great deal of money is being spent looking for bluntly toxic agents, whereas virtually no money is being spent on developing agents that spare normal cells but are toxic to one or more types of tumor.

A case in point, a reviewer for the American Cancer Society once wrote of a funding application that the "chief weakness of the proposed research is the lack of any compelling rationale for site specificity of the compound for prostatic carcinoma. In fact, the author's in vitro studies indicate that the compounds are at least as cytotoxic (and sometimes more potently) to several other types of tumor cells as the LNCaP cells."

In other words, because the proposed compound was effective against more than one type of cancer, it was considered useless. It is important to note that these comments came in spite of data that demonstrated that this compound not only led to a virtually complete eradication of prostatic tumor xenografts but also did not produce any organ-specific or other observable toxicities at doses employed. It was repeatedly stressed in this proposal that one unique property of the compound was that it was easily tolerated in vivo and therefore worthy of further investigation. Further protest and inquiry about what harm would be imposed on a patient if the potential drug is effective against more than one type of cancer—as long as it spares normal cells and tissues—met with the answer, "Our decision stands." This attitude of militant and erroneous prejudice must be changed.

Why is it necessary to bring up these points in this book, which is focused on describing the discovery and development of a new class of easily tolerated drugs? The main reason is to bring out in public what is often left unsaid in standard publications and to impress upon the reader that specificity and selectivity of drugs should be focused on sparing the host, while killing one or more types of cancer, rather than the other way around. If the drug is effective and easily tolerated, then whether it is histospecific or not is an irrelevant matter. Let's not make things more complicated than they are.

For drugs that do produce significant toxicity, histospecificity may be a more important point. By using a histospecific drug, one might expect to limit general toxicity. In reality, toxic drugs induce non-specific toxicity, often resulting in severe side effects. Chemotherapeutic drugs currently in use are highly toxic compounds and none of them meet the criteria of specificity for one tumor type as dictated by the first criterion described above. Is it not compelling enough to ask what is the purpose of this criterion after all? Obviously it has not been applied for the existing drugs, if it were then none of them should exist. Clearly the undeniable conclusion, in most generous terms, has to be that the selection process is less then fair.

Why are currently used drugs highly toxic compounds? The answer to this question is most interesting as it lies in the history of the origins of modern chemotherapy. I pause here briefly to discuss these origins before continuing with the discussion of the four remaining criteria for drug selection.

ESCAPING THE TOXICITY MODEL OF MODERN CHEMOTHERAPY

It is well documented that the effect of certain chemicals on normal tissue has been used in the discovery and development of many chemotherapeutic agents.[16] For example, in the early 1940s it was observed that nitrogen mustard (methyl-bis[chloroethyl]amine hydrochloride), a chemical warfare agent, was toxic to the normal lymphoid tissues. Further testing of this compound led to its development as an antitumor agent for lymphoid cancers. This agent caused a striking but only temporary regression of lymphoid tumors. However, toxic side effects produced by nitrogen mustard are seldom emphasized. (Incidentally, the foregoing is the most notable example cited as the origin of modern chemotherapy).[24] Similarly, in the 1960s it was observed that extract of periwinkle plant caused granulocytopenia and bone marrow suppression in normal rats. These extracts were later developed as vinca alkaloids, a new class of antitumor agent. Another example is streptozocin, a naturally occurring nitrosourea that was observed to be cytotoxic to normal pancreatic islet cells and later tested against pancreatic islet cell carcinoma. Another example of this rationale of histospecificity is the toxicity of mitotane to normal adrenal cortex that led to the development of this agent for use in adrenocortical carcinomas.

The above examples clearly demonstrate that the current criteria of drug selection can be summarized as follows. If a new compound is toxic to one or a limited number of specific normal tissue(s), then and only then might it be chosen for further development as a potential drug. This rationale of first choosing drugs that adversely affect the normal cells and tissues and then hope that the patient might live through the agony of this treatment is beyond logical comprehension. In addition, it appears that this misplaced philosophy may have assumed that "normal cells" are identical to tumor cells; a concept that is contrary to all scientific evidence. It is well established now that malignant cells or transformed cells in culture or those isolated from fresh tumor are different from normal cells in terms of their cell surface biochemistry which includes alterations in cell surface glycoproteins and glycolipids. In addition, these cells secrete tissue digesting enzymes such as proteases, collagenases and glycosidases. Tumor cells also produce altered extracellular matrix substances such as laminin and fibronectin. These cells secrete autocrine growth factors to stimulate their own growth. The rate of nucleic acid biosynthesis, as well as the levels of many other key enzymes such as topoisomerases, is higher in malignant cells as compared to normal cells. In addition, cancer cells have a variety of genetic alterations such as activated oncogenes, lack of tumor suppressor genes,[25] altered chromosomal structure, and chromosomal rearrangements. It is also becoming increasingly clear that many alterations occurring at the surface of a cancer cell are related to cell surface sugar moieties. A more common alteration in this respect is a shift to a higher molecular weight by cell surface carbohydrates caused by increased branching or increased sialylation.[26] It is these changes in the carbohydrates that have been linked with reduced cellular adhesion to extracellular matrix and with increased invasiveness and metastatic potential of malignant cells.

Thus, in my view the system of drug discovery is lopsided at best. Just imagine, if the focus of drug discovery programs would have been on finding drugs that are sparing of normal cells and tissues and toxic to one or more types of tumor cells, the current armamentarium of drugs would be quite different. Some might argue that such drugs do not exist. My answer to such pessimism is that *one is unlikely to find something that one is not looking for.* It is obvious that the issue of side effects such as diarrhea, continuous vomiting for 5 or 6 hours, hair loss, weight loss, etc. are in general more important to those who suffer from cancer. However, patients have no other choice since drugs that do not produce these effects are simply not available. This is primarily because either no one is looking for them and/or the current criteria for selecting new compounds for drug development prevents development of easily tolerated compounds.

As stated earlier, the drugs that conform to the first criterion of drug selection simply do not exist. Even so, the criterion remains on the books!

LOGIC OF CHEMOTHERAPEUTIC DOSE REVISITED

The second criterion for drug selection is the compound's potency. In this area, another misconception exists; the notion held by many scientists and physicians that if a drug is not effective at doses limited to minuscule amounts, it is useless. This rationale is based, again, on the record of toxicity of currently available drugs. Naturally, if one is using a bluntly toxic substance and hopes to have the patient live through the treatment, one has no choice but to use the compound in minute doses. Therefore, low doses are the standard. Yet, even at low doses, many of these drugs cause severe side effects. Thus, the basis for this misconception is based upon custom and experience rather than science or logic.

Why is the absolute dose considered to be so important when it is the therapeutic window of the drug that counts? If the drug is easily tolerated in gram quantities and is effective at destroying tumors, then it does not make any difference whether the drug dose is micrograms, milligrams or grams. I do not think that one has to be a scientist to understand this fundamental point requiring only common sense. Of course common sense is not so common after all.

The third criterion for drug selection is novelty of the structure of the new agent which favors selection of new agents, rather than analogs of known drugs.

The fourth criterion for drug selection aims to create what have been called "designer drugs" by identifying agents that select novel molecular targets. This is the most challenging, because it will require a more extensive characterization of the panel of 60 or more cell lines used in the screen.

The fifth criterion focuses on factors such as feasibility of synthesis and cost and availability of material, all of which could affect the selection of candidates for further development.

PHYSICIAN'S DILEMMA

A quick survey of the overall impact of the first two criteria of drug selection on new drug development could be summarized as follows. It is well documented that approximately 40 cytotoxic or antiproliferative drugs are now available for cancer therapy in United States.[16] These drugs may cure 50-75% of cancer patients predominately in the category of leukemia and lymphoma and few other relatively rare types of tumors. Only a few of these drugs have any useful clinical antitumor activity against the most common form of primary or metastatic cancer. The problem is further confounded by the fact that even tumors that are initially sensitive to a drug often rapidly become resistant to a number of other drugs in addition to the one originally used. Another major frustration encountered by most oncologists is that the available anticancer drugs as a group are monotonously similar with respect to their spectrum of clinical toxicity and mechanism of action. Most of these drugs are active primarily against actively dividing cells. Today's oncologist has to make a choice from the drugs belonging to the group of alkylating agents, antimetabolites, DNA binders, tubulin-interactive antimitotics, topoisomerase inhibitors, other agents that induce DNA strand breaks, hormones, antihormones and a few other agents with multiple or unknown mechanisms. These limitations and frustrations could at least be attenuated by allowing the development of novel drugs that do not fit the existing mold. In my opinion, the success of new drug development has been seriously hampered by these first two criteria, as they allow only the development of predominantly highly toxic agents and their analogs.

Thus, in order to improve the current armamentarium of anticancer and antiviral drugs, among other things, it is imperative that the main goal of all cancer therapy be stated for what it is, i.e. *spare the host and destroy the tumor*. This indeed should be the first criterion of drug development. The second criterion should be clearly rewritten to reflect that the quantity of the drug used for the treatment is not important as long as the patient is not harmed and the tumor is destroyed. The present criteria for drug selection must be revised. These criteria should be used as a guideline to select therapeutic agents with superior properties rather than as a cut off line. The attitude of the research community must change. And the patient—the final beneficiary of all research efforts, and who suffers the most when research misses the mark—must be heeded.

Despite the gauntlet presented by the system, in the chapters that follow we describe the discovery and development of novel chemotherapeutic agents that are not only effective against different types of malignancies and viral infections but also very sparing of the host. The process used offers an opportunity and an example for future growth and development of novel antineoplastic as well as antiviral agents.

References

1. Mathias A. The Mercurial Disease: an inquiry into the history and nature of the disease produced in the human condition by the use of mercury. 3rd ed. London: J. Callow, 1866.
2. Goldwater LJ. Mercury: a History of Quicksilver. Baltimore: York Press, 1972.
3. Hacker MP, Lazo JS, Tritton TR. Organ directed toxicities of anticancer drugs. Boston: Martinus Nijhoff Publishing, 1987.
4. Perry MC. Toxicity of chemotherapy. Semin Oncol 1982; 9:1-154.
5. Perry MC, Yarbro JW. Toxicity of chemotherapy. Orlandlo: Grune and Stratton, 1984.
6. Goldsmith MA, Slavik M, Carter SK. Quantitaive prediction of drug toxicity in humans from toxicology in small and large animals. Cancer Res 1975; 35:1354-66.
7. Driscoll JS. The preclinical new drug research program of the National Cancer Institute. Cancer Treat Rep 1984; 68:63-76.
8. Marsoni S, Hoth D, Simmon R et al. Clinical drug development: an analysis of phase II trials 1970-1985. Cancer Treat Rep 1987; 71:71-80.

9. Muggia FM. Closing the loop: providing feedback on drug development (editorial). Cancer Treat Rep 1987; 71:1-2.
10. Grindey GB. Current status of cancer drug development: failure or limited sucess. Cancer Cells 1990; 2:163-71.
11. Hamburger AW, Salmon SE. Primary bioassay of human tumor stem cells. Science 1977; 197:461-63.
12. Salmon SE, Hamburger AW, Soehnlen B et al. Quantitation of differential sensitivity of human tumor stem cells to anticancer drugs. N Eng J Med 1978; 298:1312-27.
13. Von Hoff DD, Casper J, Bradley E et al. Association between human tumor colony forming assay results and response of an individual patient's tumor to chemotherapy. Am J Med 1981; 70:1047.
14. Von Hoff DD, Clark GM, Stogdill BJ et al. Prospective clinical trial of a human tumor cloning system. Cancer Res 1983; 3:1926-31.
15. Boyd MR, Paull KD, Rubinstein LR. Data display and analysis strategies for the NCI disease-oriented in vitro antitumor drug screen. In: Valeriote FA, Corbett T, Baker L, eds. Cytotoxic anticancer drugs: models and concepts for drug discovery and development. Amsterdam: Kulwer Academic Publishers, 1992; 11-34.
16. Boyd MR. The future of new drug development. In: Niederhubr JE, ed. Current therapy in oncology. Philadelphia: BC Decker Inc., 1993; 11-22.
17. Grever MR, Hollingshead MG, Alley MC et al. Status of in vivo evaluations in the NCI anticancer drug discovery program. Proc Am Assoc Cancer Res 1994; 35:369.
18. Alley MC, Scudiero DA, Monks A et al. Feasibility of drug screening with panels of human tumor cell lines using a microculture tetrazolium assay. Cancer Res 1988; 48:589-601.
19. Rubenstein LV, Shoemaker RR, Paull KD et al. Comparision of in vitro anticancer-drug-screening. Data generated with a tetrazolium assay versus a protein assay against a diverse panel of human tumor cell lines. J Natl Cancer Inst 1990; 82:1113-18.
20. Skehan P, Storeng R, Scudiero D et al. New colorimetric cytotoxicity assay for anticancer drug screening. J Natl Cancer Inst 1990; 82:1107-12.
21. Monks A, Scudiero D, Skehan P et al. Feasibility of a high-flux anticancer drug screen utilizing a diverse panel of human tumor cell lines in culture. J Natl Cancer Inst 1991; 83:757-66.
22. Boyd MR, Paull KD. Some practical considerations and applications of the national cancer institute in vitro anticancer drug discovery screen. Drug Devel Res 1995; 34:91-109.
23. Boyd MR. Status of the NCI preclinical antitumor drug discovery screen. In: Devita VT Jr, Hellman S, Rosenberg SA, eds. Cancer: principle and practice of oncology updates. Philadelphia: JP Lippincott, 1989; 3:1-12.

24. Einhorn J. Nitrogen mustard: the origin of chemotherapy for cancer. Int J Radiat Oncol Biol Phys 1985; 11:1375-78.
25. Sager R. Tumor suppressor genes: the puzzle and the promise. Science 1989; 246:1406-10.
26. Easton EW, Bolsher, JGM, Eijnden DH. Enzymatic amplification involving glcosyltransferases from the basis for the increased size of asparagine linked glycans at the surface of NIH 3T3 cells expressing the N-ras proto-oncogenes. J Biol Chem 1991; 266:21674-80.

CHAPTER 2

Preactivation-Discovery and Biological Effects of Novel Chemotherapeutic Agents

The mind likes a strange idea as little as the body likes a strange protein, and resists it with similar energy. It would not be too fanciful to say that a new idea is the most quickly acting antigen known to science. If we watch ourselves honestly we shall often find that we have begun to argue against a new idea before it has been completely stated. —Wilfred Trotter (1872-1939) "Has the Intellect a Function?"

THE EARLY YEARS

As an immunologist, my research interests had been focused on immunotherapy of cancer involving monoclonal antibodies as a mode of drug delivery and cytokines as therapeutic agents. I had no real interest or in-depth understanding of photobiology until September 1986, when I joined the Baylor Research Foundation (now Baylor Research Institute) where several photobiology related projects were already in progress. In one of these projects lead by Dr. Lester Matthews, it was demonstrated that in vivo chloroquine resistant parasitemia caused by *P. berghei* (resistant to at least three daily doses of 0.4 mg/kg of chloroquine) could be significantly reduced when treated with hematoporphyrin derivative (HPD) prior to chloroquine injection.[1] Therefore, the following question was

Novel Chemotherapeutic Agents: Preactivation in the Treatment of Cancer and AIDS, by K. S. Gulliya.

asked; if HPD plus chloroquine = death of the parasite, then what other compound (say X) plus HPD will induce death in tumor cells? Finding the answer to this question was one of my research projects, and it involved the determination of the dark toxicity of HPD in the presence of compound X against cultured tumor cells. This was the beginning of my inculcation into the field of photodynamic therapy.

Our approach was to capitalize on the expertise of Dr. Robert Dowben in conjunction with Dr. Edward Forest, who had experience in charge transfer activities of certain compounds, having worked on the development of the photocopying process at Xerox Corporation. They provided me with a list of a number of organic compounds that should have had the best chance to elicit the combined dark toxicity of HPD for the proposed hypothesis. Unfortunately, all of the suggested compounds were found to be highly toxic to cultured cells by themselves and in combination with HPD they did not produce an enhancement of cell kill over that produced by either of the single agent alone. Thus, due to the high non-specific toxicity of a number of organic compounds tested, this project was eventually abandoned.

During this time I read papers on the photodynamic killing of malignant cells. It was clear from the limited survey of the literature that 1) photodynamic therapy with HPD was quite effective in destroying tumors; 2) sparing of the normal cells and tissue was for most part due to limiting the area of illumination to the target tumor as opposed to the property of the HPD molecule; 3) whether or not HPD was selectively retained or taken up by the tumor cells was a debatable issue; and 4) some reports claimed that higher degree of retention of HPD in tumors was due to the necrosis in the central part of the tumor and lack of circulation prevented its release from the tumor, while others denounced this concept. Thus, the mechanism of preferential accumulation of photoactive compounds into neoplastic cells was unclear. In other words, what makes a photoactive dye accumulate more in the malignant cells as compared to the normal cell? Does the interaction of the dye molecule itself with the target cell initiate certain changes in different types of cells? (It is important to note here that there are several photoactive compounds other than HPD that display a preferential affinity for tumor cells and for these compounds the mechanism of preferential affinity also remains unclear.)

These observations encouraged me to rationalize that since the first interaction of any molecule with a cell is more likely to be the plasma membrane or some structures of the plasma membrane, one logical approach would be to begin the investigation at that level. I decided to examine the possible alterations in the membrane potential of cells in response to its interaction with the photoactive compound. I learned from a paper published in Science[2] that the membrane potential of cells under certain conditions could be measured fluorometrically by using a dye called merocyanine 540. This was my introduction to this compound. Photoactive compounds are colored compounds and perhaps because of their use as coloring agents in dying of fabrics etc., they are sometimes collectively referred to as dyes. The use of the term 'dye', however, tends to invoke a feeling of something unimportant or trivial, particularly in the minds of those unfamiliar with photoreactions. Therefore, it is important to clarify that chemically speaking, photoactive agents or dyes are just like any another chemical structure whether it be aspirin or cyclophosphamide.

Further survey of the literature on cyanine dyes revealed that indeed the partition of the dye molecules between cells and extracellular medium was dependent upon membrane potential. Cell hyperpolarization (inside of the cell becomes negative) causes the dye molecules to move inside the cell whereas depolarization usually results in the release of the dye. This survey did two things for me that day. First, it was abundantly clear from the literature that the project I was intending to embark upon was significantly more complex then I had thought previously and would require dedicated efforts of biophysicists with a strong training in spectroscopy. The second and perhaps more important (even more so in retrospect) finding of the day occurred while thumbing through a current issue of *Cancer Research*, in which I noticed an article on merocyanine 540 and its use as a photodynamic agent for the purpose of autologous bone marrow purging.[3] It is very interesting to note here that during this period of time my own laboratory was in the process of being set up and I was sharing a laboratory in the bone marrow transplant unit. As a result of this association, I became more familiar with the subject of bone marrow transplantation. Thus, the paper describing the use of merocyanine 540 in bone marrow transplantation became very interesting to me due to its immediate application in the treatment of cancer, which was my major interest. The final, absolutely elating moment of the day occurred when I read that merocyanine 540 was very effective in preferentially destroying the malignant cells.

In the study published in *Cancer Research*, a 75 W GE filament light bulb (luminous flux of approx. 1170 lumens) was used as a source of white light for the in situ activation of merocyanine 540. At Baylor Research Foundation, we had access to argon lasers. Some discussions with laser physicists led us to the conclusion that lasers should be significantly better then conventional light in killing the dye-associated cancer cells. The rationale for this was based on the fact that among the prominent lines, argon laser produces a single wavelength of light at 514 nm which happens to be in the region of peak absorption for merocyanine 540. Thus, the efficiency of photon absorption at 514 nm could be expected to be significantly superior to photon absorption from a non-coherent source of light such as a light bulb. Increased efficiency of photon absorption should yield higher efficiency of tumor cell kill. In other words the difference between fluorescent light and laser light could be described by the analogy of attempting to shoot a bull's eye with a shot gun or with a rifle respectively.

Armed with this information, a number of experiments were carried out mimicking an extracorporeal model for autologous bone marrow purging. These experiments clearly demonstrated that laser light-induced photodynamic therapy with merocyanine 540 killed virtually 100% of the cancer cells and spared the majority (> 80%) of the freshly isolated normal peripheral blood mononuclear cells. These results were significantly superior to those ob-tained with the use of conventional light sources. It is important to note here that our initial experiments were carried out in the presence of fetal bovine serum. This point becomes very interesting as described below, since fetal bovine serum is unsuitable for human use.

In February 1987, I attended the proceedings of the First International Workshop on Bone Marrow Purging in Orlando, Florida. At this conference a paper on "Marrow Purging by Merocyanine 540-mediated Photolysis" was presented.[4] As an introduction to this compound, it was revealed that in the absence of serum, merocyanine 540 binds to normal as well as tumor cells without distinction. Later, during the question-answer session, Dr. Fritz Sieber stated that they were using "a special lot of pooled human AB serum" which allows them to achieve maximum selectivity between normal cells and tumor cells. Since this "special lot of serum" was not accessible to everyone, it created a serious problem. Upon my return to Dallas, we initiated screening of several different lots of human AB serum for their effect on providing protection to the normal cells and allowing the killing of cultured tumor cells. To our disappointment, we found that in the presence of human AB serum the killing of cancer cells was reduced and killing of normal cells was increased. This was a serious setback to say the least, because one could essentially spend a lifetime in search of "a special lot of human serum." Thus, this approach was abandoned and tests on human albumin, a major component of serum, were initiated. This factor was most important if this system were ever going to be considered for clinical use.

Later through trial and error we learned that 2.5% of human albumin produced best results, as it protected up to 85% of the normal cells and allowed killing 4-6 logs of leukemia and lymphoma cells when illuminated in the presence of merocyanine 540. A very brief summary of this experience regarding our findings with human AB serum and human albumin was later published.[5] Thus, through these research efforts we demonstrated that one optimal condition for using merocyanine 540 in conventional photodynamic therapy in terms of maximizing tumor cell kill and sparing of normal cells was the use of human albumin. In addition, we were the first to use laser irradiation for the purpose of autologous bone marrow purging, which minimized the non-specific toxicity of light and increased tumor cell kill (light from conventional sources has been reported to kill over 60% of certain types of cells). By using these perimeters we were able to demonstrate that selective killing of certain types of tumor cells was easily achieved.[5-7]

During the course of this research we also demonstrated that certain tumor cells, e.g. lung adenocarcinoma and breast cancer cells which previously were reported to be resistant to merocyanine 540 plus white light-induced photolysis,[3] were quite easily destroyed when laser light was employed[8,9] instead of the white light from fluorescent bulbs.

Experiments designed to enhance our understanding of the underlying mechanisms of preferential phototoxicity of merocyanine 540 towards certain types of cancer cells were carried out in collaboration with Dr. Anthony Harriman, Center for Fast Kinetics

Research, University of Texas at Austin. This work, described in detail in chapter 3, was also instrumental in delineating the photoreactions involved in the process of preactivation.

DISCOVERY OF PREACTIVATION

Research work related to bone marrow purging continued for a couple of years. Among the two most important findings were 1) that the effect of light alone is not as insignificant as generally reported in the literature and therefore should not be ignored; and 2) the dark toxicity or non-specific toxicity of many dyes including hematoporphyrin derivative or photofrin II is also quite significant and must be taken into account.

Thus, with the first hand knowledge that each agent (photoactive compound and light) is independently causing a significant effect, it was very difficult for me to design an experiment that would produce a meaningful answer to any questions related to the mechanism of action of preferential tumor cell killing effect. This is because one of the fundamental tenets of all scientific research is that one must study one variable at a time. Pondering these limitations and how to transform a two variable system into a one variable system, it occurred to me that if the photoactive compound was first illuminated with light and then mixed with tumor cells, it would then be possible to reduce the aforementioned two variable system to a one variable system. Since I did not have formal training in the field of photobiology, it did not occur to me that 1) the idea was against an established principle of photobiology; and 2) as I later found out, everyone in this field that I talked to thought that it would never work. Fortunately, we consulted the gurus after the fact. We had no idea at the time that this process would create multiple photoproducts, and later as it turns out, they were isolated, characterized and chemically synthesized. Indeed these experiments were carried out and photoproducts thus produced were successful in the killing of tumor cells and sparing of normal cells. This was the birth of "preactivation," a term we coined approximately 10 or 11 months after the fact, to distinguish it from conventional photodynamic therapy for the purposes of patent protection.

Thus, the process of preactivation of photoactive compounds was discovered in 1989. This process utilizes a principle of photodynamic therapy and leads to production of novel photoproducts that mediate their biological effects *independent* of light. Since photoactive compounds as well as a principle of photodynamic therapy are involved, a very brief overview of photodynamic therapy and one of its major limitations is first described. Exhaustive discussion or references for photodynamic therapy are not provided as many books and numerous papers in this field are easily available.

The "ideal goal" for the treatment of cancer, and for that matter any disease, is that the therapeutic agent must spare the normal cells and tissues (host) and destroy the malignancy or disease-causing organism. This condition is of paramount importance, because otherwise the host (patient) will be killed either by the disease or by the treatment. When a therapeutic agent meets this "ideal" requirement but only in parts or different degrees, side effects are produced. Side effects such as nausea, vomiting, hair loss, etc. are the manifestations of the impaired functions of normal cells and tissues. A vast majority of currently available anticancer treatments produce severe side effects and the patient has no choice except to refuse the treatment because drugs that are easily tolerated, i.e. produce minimal if any side effects, have not been discovered. Therefore, there is a constant need for the development of new and improved effective drugs that are easily tolerated. The term "easily tolerated" is carefully employed in the previous statement because drugs with zero side effects do not exist. Does that mean that the ideal goal (i.e. zero side effects) for treatment cannot be met? In the strictest sense the answer is 'no' because even easily tolerated drugs will perturb the normal system even though the effects may be too minuscule to be perceived. One way of approaching the ideal goal is by using drugs that spare the normal cells but interact with the abnormal or malignant cells. This property sometimes is an inherent characteristic of the drug molecule, while at other times it can be manipulated by employing target-specific delivery agents such as monoclonal antibodies. Many photoactive compounds, however, display an inherent preferential affinity for certain types of tumors. The selectivity of such a photoactive compound is further enhanced by illumination of only the target site since the lethal photochemical reaction ensues only after its illumination. Thus, photoactive dyes have been used as antitumor agents. Tumor cells containing photoactive dyes are killed upon exposure to light.

WHAT EVERY STUDENT OF PHOTODYNAMIC THERAPY SHOULD KNOW

Photosensitizers combined with light exposure are one of the oldest treatments known. They have been used by ancient Egyptians and Indians who ingested *Ammi majus*, a plant rich in psoralens, followed by sun bathing for the treatment of vitiligo, leprosy and other skin disorders. In 1903, Von Tappeiner used eosin plus light to treat skin cancer, cutaneous lupus and condyloma latum. In 1913, Meyer-Betz injected himself with hematoporphyrin and demonstrated its potency by suffering from photosensitivity for several months. In the 1960s, a crude derivative of hematoporphyrin was shown to localize and photosensitize animal tumors. In 1978, Dougherty and colleagues demonstrated that this hematoporphyrin derivative could be administered intravenously and when followed by red light exposure, caused a partial or complete clinical response in a variety of human tumors. Now, photodynamic therapy (PDT) has gained significant acceptance in the clinic and is under intense investigation around the world, not only for the irradication of solid tumors but also for the extracorporeal purging of contaminated blood, blood products and for skin disorders. Many different dyes have been proposed and in particular, porphyrin and phthalocyanine derivatives are extremely popular materials. This subject has attracted the attention of synthetic chemists, who are actively engaged in designing new dyes which absorb at long wavelengths since longer wavelengths of light penetrate deeper into the target tissue.[10] The main role of the photochemists has been to identify dyes which possess high triplet state quantum yields[11,12] and which generate singlet oxygen in high yield upon irradiation in O_2-saturated solution. Dyes which meet these criteria are designated as potential PDT sensitizers, and dyes that do not produce significant yields of singlet oxygen have received no further attention because singlet oxygen is believed to be the sole cytotoxic agent.[13,14] However, this does not appear to be the case since the involvement of singlet oxygen in actual PDT processes is plausible, and in certain cases highly likely, but completely unproven and there is not always a correlation between the observed cytotoxicity and yield of singlet oxygen.[15]

In addition to these unresolved fundamental issues, a serious limitation of photodynamic therapy has been stated to be that "it can only be effective at sites where light can penetrate, such as the oral cavity, the bladder, the lower genitourinary tract, lungs and any surface approachable by fiber optics."[16] The target tumor has to be large enough to be visible to the naked eye. Therefore, the metastatic involvement of lymph nodes or circulating metastatic cells or viral infections would make photodynamic therapy unlikely to be successful because not only is the target too small to be visible to the naked eye, but it is only a matter of time before the malignant tumor reappears or it may already be in the process of formation at a distant site.

One of the most important points to remember is that treatment of malignant cancer is essentially the treatment of metastases and anything that falls short of this requirement is incomplete. At present, PDT can only be used for the elimination of a specific tumor and not the renegade tumor cells or metastasis, i.e. cancer as a disease. Therefore, it would be ideal if photoactive compounds could be made to exert their cytotoxic effects independent of light. If successful, this development would eliminate the major limitation of photodynamic therapy (described above), and may lead to the treatment of viral infections and malignancies that otherwise could not be treated with conventional photodynamic therapy alone.

THE HYPOTHESIS OF LIGHT-ACTIVATED INTERMEDIATES (PREACTIVATION)

In view of the single variable approach accomplished in pilot experiments by the pre-illumination of merocyanine 540 and its subsequent success in killing of tumor cells independent of light, we postulated that this phenomenon might involve a light-activated intermediate. In addition, this metastable active intermediate might be sufficiently long lived so that the irradiation of the dye and the killing of the cells eventually could be separated in time. Therefore, a series of systematic experiments were performed in which a solution of photoactive dye merocyanine 540 was first irradiated (preactivated) with argon laser light and the resultant mixture of photoproducts (pMC540) were allowed to interact with cultured tumor cells. A significant killing of tumor cells was observed, thereby proving our hypothesis. A description of experiments that led to further development of preactivation technology is presented.

TERMINOLOGY USED

As stated earlier, the term "preactivation" was coined to distinguish this process of photoproduct generation from conventional photodynamic therapy. Other terms such as pre-illumination, pre-irradiation, light-exposed and photoproducts have been used interchangeably by the researchers in the field. However, the term photoproducts (used for a very long time) unless clearly specified, can also refer to those formed in situ under conventional photodynamic therapy. In this book, however, the term "photoproducts" unless otherwise specified, has been used exclusively to describe the photocleavage products formed under the process of preactivation.

In recent literature involving photodynamic therapy, disclaimer statements that "photoproducts were ineffective," i.e. photoproducts produced by using the process of preactivation were found to be ineffective, have appeared. These conclusions, however, should be viewed with a great deal of caution because both inactive and active photoproducts can be produced depending upon the conditions employed. Therefore, the involvement of photoproducts during conventional PDT can only be proved by systematic analysis of all associated perimeters which as of this writing has not been reported in the literature. Thus, the crucial remaining task for those in the field of PDT who continue to subscribe to the notion that singlet oxygen generated at triplet state is the sole causative agent of cytotoxicity is to prove that photoproducts are not involved. Simply irradiating a dye solution under the conditions used for conventional PDT and then allowing the irradiated dye to interact with the tumor cells to determine whether photoproducts were involved in the PDT process or not may be a good starting point but it is not sufficient. This is because during the irradiation procedure of conventional PDT, active photoproducts may have been formed well before the termination point of the experiment and could have interacted with the cells rapidly. Thus, to allow for the aforementioned possibility one must conduct a well-defined systematic study in which a dye solution is exposed to light for different periods of time followed by a biological evaluation of the resultant products in a manner required for developing a time course and drug dose responses.

IS PREACTIVATION REAL?

The first few experiments involving pre-illumination (preactivation) of photoactive compounds were exciting because the treatment of cultured tumor cells with the preactivated compound produced a significant killing of the tumor cells in the absence of direct illumination. However, there were many unanswered questions regarding the validity of the process of preactivation because it was not supposed to have worked. For example, is the process of preactivation creating toxic products from the solvent used to solubilize the compound? Is the heat produced during the irradiation process responsible for the generation of toxic entities? Is it reproducible? Is the application of the process limited to only one photoactive compound, i.e. merocyanine 540? Is the preactivated material stable? If so, for how long? Even though these thoughts and comments encountered at the time were eventually examined, a major source of confidence against these types of questions stemmed from our initial experiment in which it was observed that preactivated merocyanine 540 spared the majority of fresh human peripheral blood mononuclear cells. These results were virtually identical to those obtained under conventional photodynamic therapy using merocyanine 540. Thus, it was clear that even though the process of preactivation causes a major change in the structure of the original compound, the resultant mixture of new compounds retained many of the original properties. In addition, even if one considers that the toxic products produced were arising from a nonspecific process, it is unlikely that they would display a preferential affinity towards malignant cells.

Nonetheless, a number of control experiments were done to answer questions related to the validity of preactivation. Results from some of the key experiments are summarized below.

1) The process of preactivation was applicable to a variety of an unrelated class of photoactive compounds such as hematoporphyrin derivative,[17] carbocyanines and many derivatives of these compounds. Therefore, we concluded that preactivation was not limited to merocyanine 540 alone.
2) Photoproducts thus produced are stable for a relatively long period of time. For example, preactivated merocyanine 540 could be stored at low temperature for a month,[18] without significant loss in in vitro cytotoxicity.

3) Preactivation of dye solvent or culture medium alone did not produce toxicity in cultured tumor cells, indicating that the observed cytotoxic effects were not due to some non-specific action of light on the components of solvent or growth medium used.
4) Photoproducts could not be generated by the application of heat or alteration of pH of the dye solution.
5) Preactivation of dry photoactive compound was unsuccessful.

It is important to note that optimal conditions required for preactivation of a given photoactive compound are expected to be different requiring a systematic search for the appropriate combination of duration and intensity of light irradiation. This arbitrary search process for optimal conditions could be simplified by using the in vitro conditions employed for conventional PDT. For example, from our in vitro conventional photodynamic therapy experiments, we knew that a mixture of tumor cells plus MC540 [20 μg/ml (35.1μM)] when irradiated with 93.6 J/cm^2 of 514 nm argon laser light, produced a 99.99% tumor cell kill. Therefore, for our initial preactivation experiments, we simply employed these conditions except tumor cells were left out. In addition, these experiments also suggest that virtually identical photoproducts may be emerging under the conditions of conventional PDT. However, a comparison of the identity of photoproducts generated under the conditions of PDT and preactivation remains to be done. This task will be complex because under the condition of PDT the ensuing photoproduct may react rapidly with the available biological target yielding a different end product. In any event, the fact that stable cytotoxic photoproducts are formed under preactivation conditions demonstrates that the role of singlet oxygen produced at excited states at least in the case of merocyanine 540 has more to do with the production of photoproducts than the actual cell kill. Studies of the photochemistry and photophysics of merocyanine 540 (chapter 3) clearly demonstrate that this indeed is the case.

More recently, photoproducts generated upon pre-illumination of merocyanine 540 and their role in subsequent dark toxicity[19] as well as photoproducts generated from other pre-illuminated photoactive compounds in simple solutions has been reported by other researchers in the field.[20-22]

PROCESS OF PREACTIVATION

A stock solution of merocyanine 540 (1 mg/ml) can be preactivated by irradiation with 514 nm argon laser light for one hour set at 4 watts. Later we discovered that virtually identical results are obtained by employing a bank of fluorescent lights for a period of 18 hours. There is no significant difference in the observed cytotoxicity or absorption spectrum of pMC540 obtained from either of these two methods. During irradiation, there is a time dependent progressive color change in the dye solution which is indicative of a continuous chemical reaction underway. In other words photoproducts are probably continuously being formed and it is imperative that photoreaction be terminated at a certain optimal point in order to obtain a useful product. The termination point, of course will depend on the nature of the photoactive compound, wavelength(s) and intensity of light used (if light is the activating agent), temperature, oxygen and the duration of illumination. All these variables have the potential to drive the photochemical reaction along possibly several different pathways and thus must be controlled tightly for a given purpose. For example, under the uncontrolled conditions of continuous pre-illumination of merocyanine 540, the reaction can be driven to a point where the dye is completely bleached. In this state pMC540 is non-toxic to the cultured neoplastic cells.

OTHER SOURCES OF ENERGY FOR PREACTIVATION

In principle, any electromagnetic source emitting energy in the region of the absorption spectrum of a chromophore containing compound can be used for the purpose of preactivation. We have successfully used light from a free electron laser source for preactivation of merocyanine 540. In addition, gamma radiation from a cobalt source was also successful for this purpose. However, a detailed characterization of the perimeters required for optimal photoproduct generation from these energy sources remains to be done.

PREACTIVATION OF OTHER CLASSES OF PHOTOACTIVE COMPOUNDS

As mentioned earlier, the process of preactivation is applicable to virtually all photoactive compounds. However, whether a useful photoproduct will be produced or not is a separate issue. The following photoactive compounds have been successfully preactivated to produce cytotoxic photoproducts displaying a degree of preferential affinity for certain types of malignant cells in our laboratory: certain cyanines and carbocyanines, several analogs of merocyanine, hematoporphyrin derivatives,[17] benzoporphyrin, extended ring porphyrins and rhodamine 123. From these results it is clear that preactivation is not limited to a specific class of photoactive compounds.

PHYSICAL PROPERTIES OF PREACTIVATED MEROCYANINE 540 (pMC540)

During preactivation, one of the most obvious changes is the change in the color of the compound. The original dark reddish-brown color of merocyanine 540 is altered to a pale yellow color with a brownish tint when it is converted into preactivated merocyanine 540 (pMC540). A more definitive and quantitative measure of this change is the shift in the absorption maxima from 533 nm to 280 nm (Fig. 2.1).

Analysis of pMC540 by reverse phase high pressure liquid chromatography revealed a number of distinct peaks (Fig. 2.2). The chromatographic profile could be divided into three separate regions. Three major areas could also be resolved when the separation of photoproducts from pMC540 is carried out by thin layer chromatography. Fast atom bombardment mass spectrometry and NMR analysis of the non-activated and preactivated compound also revealed a significant difference between these two compounds. From these studies it was concluded that pMC540 is significantly different from the parent compound, which appears to have been cleaved to form new compounds.

Later, three photoproducts, meroxazole, merocil and merodantoin (Fig. 2.3) were isolated and characterized by Franck et al.[23] Their chemical syntheses have been worked out. As will be described later, only merocil and merodantoin are the biologically active photoproducts which produce cytotoxicities higher than or comparable to the mixture of photoproducts in pMC540 (chapters 4 and 5). All data presented in this book were obtained by using pMC540 as well as its chemically synthesized isolates merocil and merodantoin. It is important to note here that part of in vitro data related to merocil and merodantoin appears in chapters 4 and

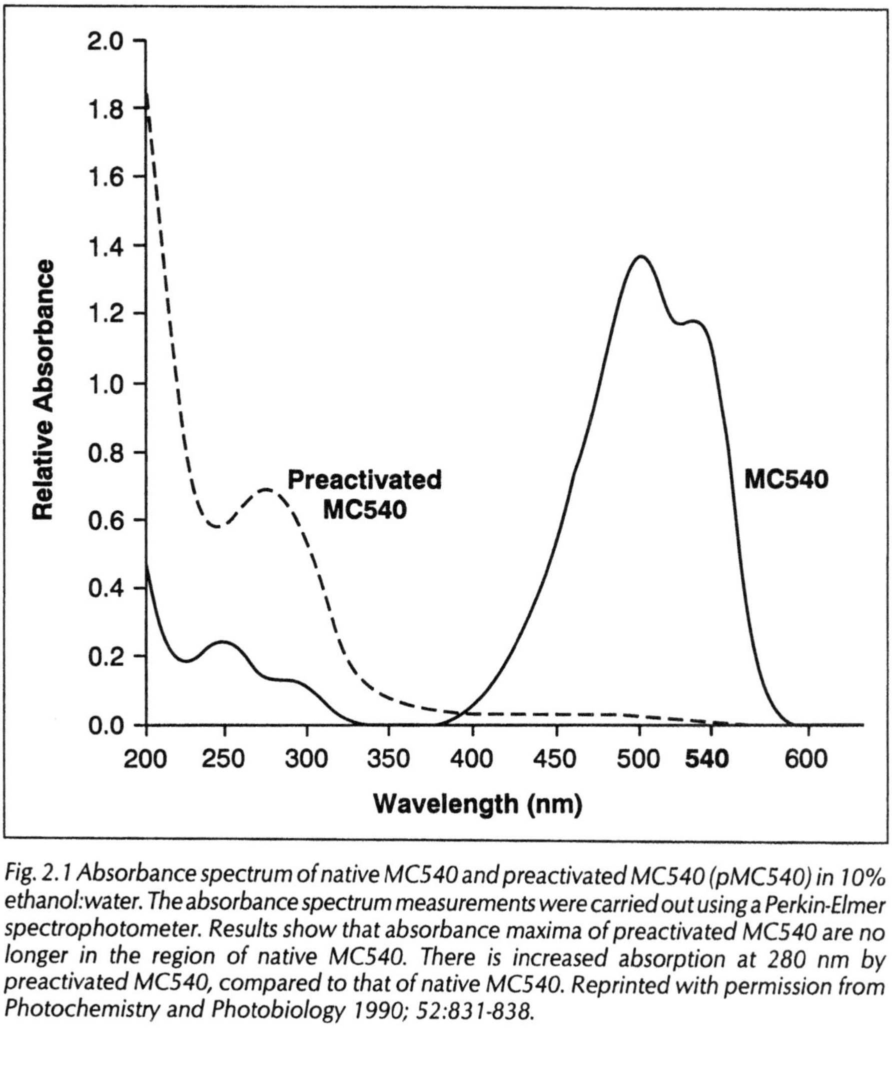

Fig. 2.1 Absorbance spectrum of native MC540 and preactivated MC540 (pMC540) in 10% ethanol:water. The absorbance spectrum measurements were carried out using a Perkin-Elmer spectrophotometer. Results show that absorbance maxima of preactivated MC540 are no longer in the region of native MC540. There is increased absorption at 280 nm by preactivated MC540, compared to that of native MC540. Reprinted with permission from Photochemistry and Photobiology 1990; 52:831-838.

5 as it establishes the rationale and background for studies described in these chapters.

Stability of Preactivated MC540

Determinations of the stability of preactivated merocyanine 540 (pMC540) revealed that this product was stable for a week at room temperature and a month at -75° C or -135° C as judged by cytotoxicity assays (Table 2.1). When pMC540 was heated to 42° C for one hour, only 20% of the toxicity towards cultured Daudi cells was lost. Because pMC540 is a mixture of photoproducts, analysis of changes in the chemical composition could not be

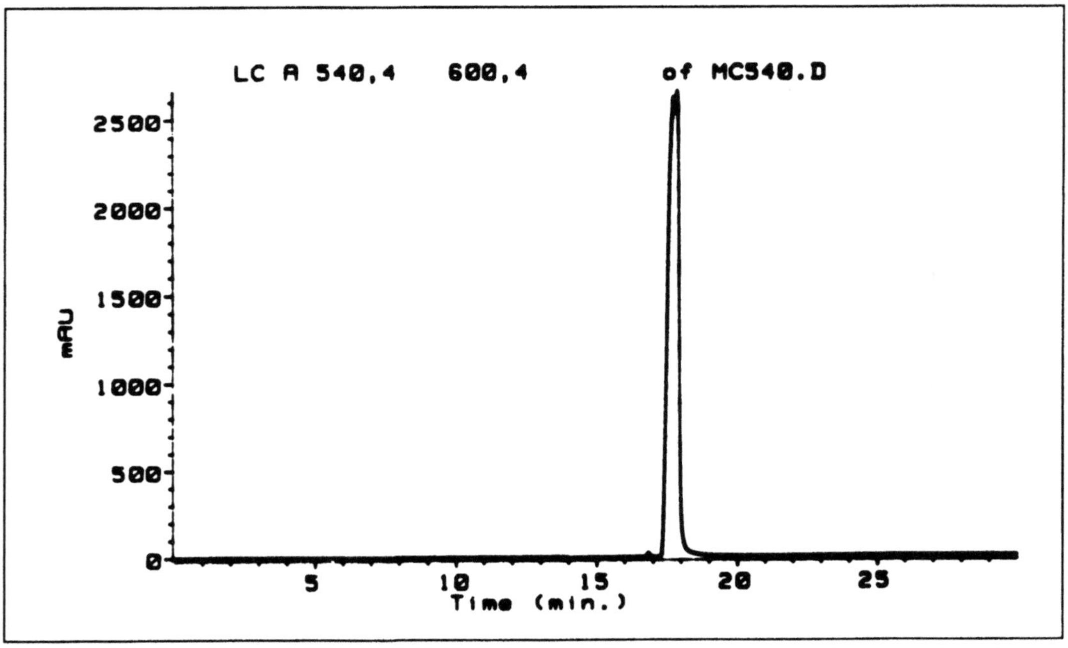

Fig. 2.2a.

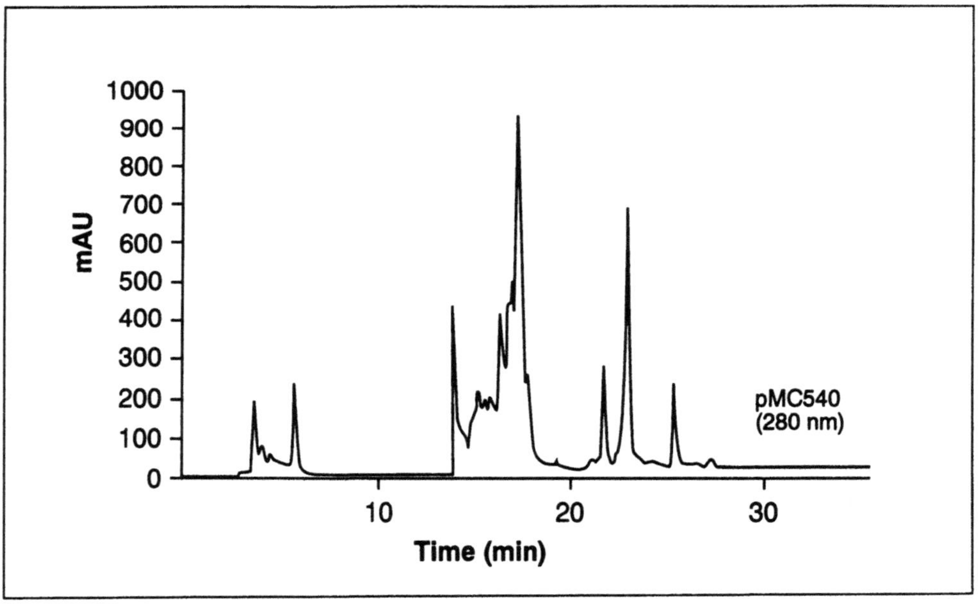

Fig. 2.2b.

Fig. 2.2 HPLC analysis of native MC540 (a, top) and preactivated MC540 (b, bottom). The elution profile of preactivated MC540 is different from that of native MC540, indicating that preactivated MC540 is significantly different than the parent compound. A detection wavelength of 540 nm was used for native MC540, while 280 nm was used for preactivated MC540 because its elution profile was undetectable at 540 nm. Reprinted with permisssion from Photochemistry and Photobiology 1990; 2:831-838.

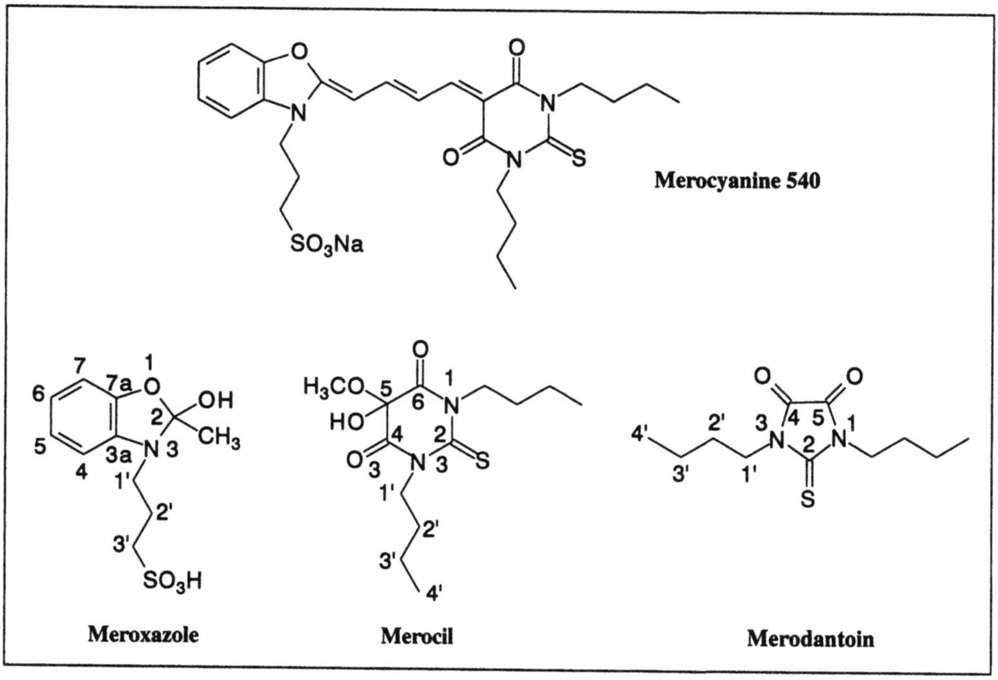

Fig. 2.3. Structures of native merocyanine 540 and three photoproducts, meroxazole, merocil and merodantoin, isolated from preactivated merocyanine 540. Reprinted with permission from Anticancer Drugs 1994; 5:557-566.

Table 2.1. Stability of preactivated merocyanine 540 at various temperatures

Storage Temperature	Number of Days Stored	Cytotoxicity† (%)
25°C	Fresh	100
42°C (1 hour)	Fresh	80
25°C	1	95
25°C	2	94
25°C	3	91
-10°C	7	89
-10°C	15	84
-10°C	30	80
-135°C	7	93
-135°C	15	90
-135°C	30	91
-135°C	180	65

†The cytotoxity of freshly prepared preactivated merocyanine 540 (pMC540) was determined on HL-60 target cells by trypan blue dye exclusion method. The cytotoxicity was calculated as a percentage of control (fresh). All experiments were repeated at least three times. Reprinted with permisssion from Photochemistry and Photobiology 1990; 2:831-838.

performed for determinations of the structural stability of the compound. However, later purified photoproducts merocil and merodantoin, as well as their chemically synthesized forms, were obtained and found to be quite stable at room temperature for more than one year.

Dose of pMC540

The dose of pMC540 used in all studies reported to date is identical to the initial concentration of non-activated merocyanine 540 used for preactivation. For example, 10 μg/ml (17.55 μM) of non-activated merocyanine 540 would yield 10 μg/ml (17.55 μM) of pMC540.

In Vitro Cytotoxicity of Preactivated MC540

Since in preliminary studies it was determined that tumor cell kill could be obtained by using the photoproducts in the absence of light, the first set of experiments was designed to assess the selectivity of pMC540 towards malignant cells. For this purpose the cytotoxicity of pMC540 against a panel of cultured tumor cells obtained from a variety of human and rodent cell lines was used. Human peripheral blood mononuclear cells isolated from freshly donated blood obtained from healthy volunteers were used as a source of normal cells. Results from these experiments clearly indicated that pMC540 is cytotoxic to certain types (but not all) of cancer cells, whereas the normal cells remained virtually unaffected (Table 2.2). Human leukemia HL-60, lymphoma Daudi, breast cancers MCF-7 and BT-20, small cell lung carcinoma H-69 and prostate cancers DU145 were among the most susceptible cancer types whereas multiple myeloma ARH77, lung carcinoma A549 and malignant melanoma G361 cells were not affected at all. These data clearly demonstrated that pMC540 was not a general toxin.

Later we discovered that the preferential affinity of pMC540 was not restricted to only malignant cells but it also included activated, transformed virus-infected cells and cell-free enveloped viruses. However, a majority (85%) of normal mature cells were not affected at a dose that killed 90% of the malignant cells. These data were obtained under the condition of a 24 hour continuous drug exposure of the target cells.[18,24] Subsequent experiments (Fig. 2.4) revealed that by increasing the duration of treatment from 24 hours to 72 hours the dose of pMC540 could be reduced from

120 μg/ml (210.6 μM) to 4.5 μg/ml (7.9 μM) to obtain a 90% killing of human lymphoma Daudi cells. Similar results were obtained when the drug was removed after 6 hours of incubation by washing, and cells were further incubated for 72 hours. Taken together, these results suggest that after the initial lethal hit a prolonged period of time was required for cell death to occur.

Table 2.2. Comparative dark cytotoxicity of native MC540 and preactivated MC540*

Cell Type	Cell Origin	Dose (μg/ml)	Native MC540	Preactivated MC540	p-Value
Peripheral Blood Lymphocyte	Normal Human Blood	40	8.4 ± 5.6	6.77 ± 2.54	> 0.1
		80	12 ± 4.8	8.30 ± 3.21	< 0.1
		120	Not Done	15.00 ± 5.80	
Daudi	Human Burkitt Lymphoma	40	12.55 ± 3.18	51.79 ± 5.07	< .005
		80	40.10 ± 1.83	88.80 ± 12.11	< .01
		120	58.15 ± 7.99	89.99 ± 15.51	< .05
HL-60	Human Leukemia	40	22.28 ± 5.51	53.86 ± 4.52	< .005
		80	31.66 ± 3.02	65.66 ± 10.34	< .025
		120	64.04 ± 6.67	87.93 ± 4.87	< .01
L1210	Murine Leukemia	40	14.05 ± 1.76	51.10 ± 4.96	< .005
		80	50.50 ± 2.68	63.00 ± 6.16	< .05
		120	57.55 ± 5.30	86.87 ± 6.38	< .01
HS-Sultan	Human Multiple Myeloma	40	9.40 ± 1.13	29.86 ± 6.07	< .025
		80	32.65 ± 4.73	56.26 ± 8.55	< .025
		120	47.00 ± 4.00	70.60 ± 5.19	< .01
GM-1312	Human Multiple Myeloma	40	10.35 ± 3.46	42.66 ± 8.08	< .01
		80	32.50 ± 2.17	65.33 ± 12.01	< .025
		120	51.05 ± 1.77	77.00 ± 8.18	< .025
H-69	Human Small Cell Lung Carcinoma	40	10.60 ± 4.80	45.11 ± 9.28	< .025
		80	25.60 ± 5.94	57.36 ± 6.50	< .01
		120	48.00 ± 5.94	88.56 ± 3.56	< .005

*Preactivated MC540 (pMC540) was obtained as follows: A solution of native MC540 (1mg/ml; 10% ethanol:H_2O) was irradiated with 514 nm laser light, set at four watts for one hour. This preparation was used immediately. Except for the preparation of preactivated MC540, all experiments were carried out in the dark. Data shown is percent inhibition (mean ± S.D.) of ^{3}H-Thymidine uptake by dye-treated cells calculated as a percentage of untreated controls. Doses of pMC540 used were 40 μg/ml (70.2 μM); 80 μg/ml (140.4 μM); 120 μg/ml (210.6 μM). Reprinted with permisssion from Photochemistry and Photobiology 1990; 2:831-838.

Fig. 2.4 Human lymphoma Daudi cells (1 x 10⁴ cells/ml) were treated under the conditions of continuous exposure with either vehicle (control), or preactivated merocyanine 540 [1.4 μg/ml (2.46 μM) or 4.3 μg/ml (7.9 μM)]. Viability of cells was determined by trypan blue dye exclusion method on indicated days.

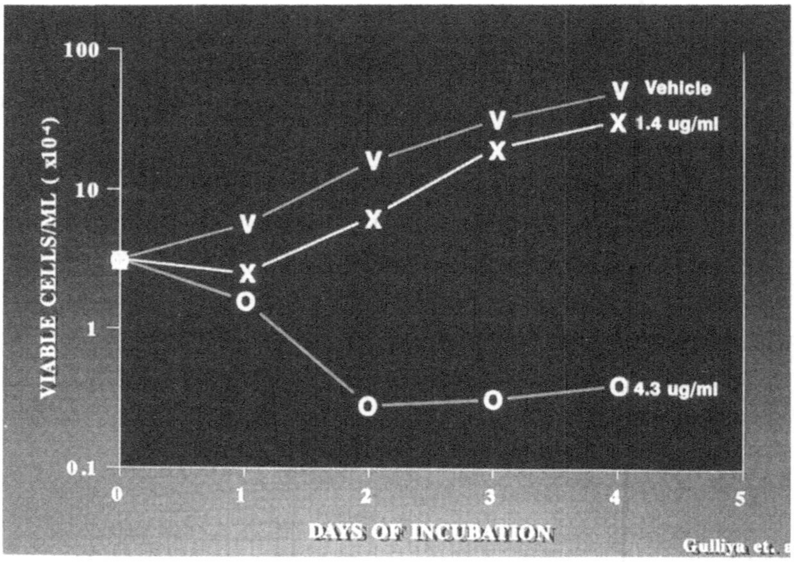

Next, effects of pMC540 on the colonogenic growth of cultured tumor cells from different cell lines were also determined by using a colony formation assay. For this purpose cells were treated with either pMC540, non-activated MC540, or left untreated. After 24 hours of incubation 2 x 10^5 cells were plated in culture plates containing 1 ml of 0.8% methylcellulose, 20% fetal bovine serum, 0.6 mM 2-mercaptoethanol and 100 units of penicillin/100 μg streptomycin. Colonies consisting of 50 or more cells were counted on day 7. Results from these experiments show (Table 2.3) that pMC540 treatment even at a sub-lethal in vitro dose of 80 μg/ml caused a significant inhibition of colonogenic growth. These data support the effectiveness of pMC540.

In yet another set of experiments, effects of pMC540 and merodantoin (one of the most active chemically synthesized isolates from pMC540) on a panel of breast cancer cell lines was investigated. In these experiments breast cancer cells were treated with different doses of pMC540 and merodantoin for a period of 24 hours to 96 hours. After each incubation period cell kill was determined by MTT assay. Results from these experiments are shown in Tables 2.4 and 2.5. It is clear from the data presented that breast ductal carcinoma T47D and BT474 cells were susceptible to the cytotoxic action of pMC540 and cell kill was dose and time dependent. All cell lines tested were susceptible to the cytotoxic action of merodantoin producing approximately 90% cell kill at a dose of 48 μg/ml (198.24 μM). The most sensitive cell lines in this group were MB436 followed by MCF-7 requiring 15 μg/ml (61.95 μM) and 25 μg/ml (103.25 μM) of drug to produce a 90% cell kill.

Table 2.3. Effect of native and preactivated MC540 on the survival of clonogenic tumor stem cells from various cell lines

Cell Lines	Number of Colonies (mean ± S.D.) Untreated	Native MC540 (80 μg/ml))	Preactivated MC540 (80 μg/ml)	p-Value†
HL-60	533.33 ± 61.10	378.00 ± 49.48	166.66 ± 12.11	< .001
Daudi	622.66 ± 51.59	368.33 ± 44.41	101.33 ± 22.03	< .001
H-69	488.33 ± 28.43	328.00 ± 33.06	174.00 ± 36.09	< .01
L1210	426.66 ± 16.65	295.00 ± 28.48	147.00 ± 17.52	< .005

†The cytotoxicity of preactivated MC540 is significantly (as shown by p-values) higher than the native MC540. 80 μg/ml = 140.4 μM

Table 2.4 Effect of preactivated MC540 on breast cancer cell lines

Cell Type	**pMC540 (μg/ml)**	**Percentage Cell Kill (mean ± S.D.)** 24 Hours	48 Hours	72 Hours	96 Hours
T47D, ductal carcinoma	40	3	8	12	62.3 ± 9.7
	80	16	5	15	93.0 ± 4.0
	120	22	11	33	94.0 ± 4.4
BT474, ductal carcinoma	40	0	1	7	17.0 ± 5.6
	80	13	1	6	66 ± 6.2
	120	14	11	15	80.7 ± 1.0
MB231, breast adenocarcinoma	40	0 ± 0	1.0 ± 1.0	5.0 ± 1.0	1.0 ± 2.3
	80	0 ± 0	1.7 ± 2.1	8.0 ± 1.7	2.4 ± 4.8
	120	0.33 ± 0.58	7.0 ± 6.1	8.0 ± 0	4.4 ± 5.9
MB436, breast adenocarcinoma	40	0 ± 0	4.7 ± 4.5	5.0 ± 8.7	0 ± 0
	80	0 ± 0	0 ± 0	0 ± 0	0 ± 0
	120	0 ± 0	0 ± 0	0 ± 0	0 ± 0
MB453, Breast carcinoma	40	3.0 ± 3.0	3.0 ± 3.6	13.0 ± 3.6	0.33 ± 0.58
	80	3.67 ± 1.2	2.0 ± 1.7	13.3 ± 2.9	0.67 ± 0.58
	120	3.3 ± 1.2	9.7 ± 1.5	15.3 ± 2.1	1.7 ± 1.5

Dose of pMC540: 40 μg/ml (70.2 μM); 80 μg/ml (140.4 μM); 120 μg/ml (210.6 μM).

ACTIVITY OF pMC540 AND MERODANTOIN IN A HUMAN TUMOR CLONING ASSAY

It is clear from the data presented thus far that both pMC540 and merodantoin display preferential cytotoxicity to certain types of cultured tumor cells. Encouraged by these results we elected to

Table 2.5 Effect of merodantoin on breast cancer cell lines

Cell Type	Merodantoin (μg/ml)	Percentage Cell Kill (Mean ± S.D.) 24 Hours	48 Hours	72 Hours	96 Hours
T47D, ductal carcinoma	6				32.7 ± 4.0
	12	43	50	70	52.3 ± 4.0
	24	35	48	71	69.0 ± 13.0
	36				79.0 ± 11.4
	48				90.0 ± 7.8
	60				92.0 ± 4.4
BT474, ductal carcinoma	6				28.3 ± 1.0
	12	16	17	49	43.7 ± 4.5
	24	25	44	67	64.7 ± 3.5
	36				80.0 ± 2.6
	48				91.7 ± 3.5
	60				91.7 ± 3.2
MB231, breast adenocarcinoma	6	18.7 ± 8.1	42.0 ± 6.2	37.7 ± 2.1	7 ± 2.6
	12	36.0 ± 7.5	71.3 ± 0.58	68.7 ± 2.1	24.3 ± 2.1
	24	52.0 ± 9.5	81.0 ± 6.9	73.7 ± 0.58	62.0 ± 2.6
	36	52.3 ± 13.6	95.3 ± 2.1	90.3 ± 2.5	87.0 ± 2.6
	48	83.3 ± 12.5	94.3 ± 1.5	93.7 ± 1.5	93.0 ± 1.0
	60	68.3 ± 6.5	95.0 ± 4.0	94.0 ± 1.0	97.3 ± 1.5
MB436, breast adenocarcinoma	1	21.3 ± 15	17.7 ± 6.8	15.7 ± 7.4	26.7 ± 13
	5	40.7 ± 13	41.7 ± 11	50 ± 12	54.7 ± 10
	10	43 ± 7.0	60 ± 6.2	63.7 ± 11	74 ± 6.0
	15	50 ± 12	64 ± 8.7	75.7 ± 6.7	89 ± 6.2
	25	71 ± 15	82.7 ± 7.4	91.3 ± 8.1	95.7 ± 4.0
	35	74.7 ± 18	87.7 ± 5.5	89.3 ± 11	94.7 ± 4.7
MB453, breast carcinoma	6	12.0 ± 2.6	8.0 ± 3.0	10.7 ± 7.1	1.7 ± 2.9
	12	42.3 ± 2.1	59.0 ± 1.7	57.0 ± 3.6	5.0 ± 3.0
	24	69.7 ± 7.0	66.3 ± 2.1	72.3 ± 1.5	51.7 ± 5.1
	36	68.0 ± 2.0	97.0 ± 1.0	96.0 ± 1.7	96.0 ± 1.0
	48	90.7 ± 1.5	97.0 ± 1.0	96.7 ± 0.6	96.7 ± 0.6
	60	90.0 ± 3.0	96.7 ± 1.5	96.3 ± 1.2	96.7 ± 1.5

Merodantoin dose: 1 μg/ml = 4.13 μM

determine their effect on human tumor colony forming units. This assay, as described in chapter 1 of this book, is one of the three tests used in the screening of new drugs for further research and development. A key feature of this test is that it utilizes fresh human tumors taken directly from patients and then cultured in soft agar. Published literature on this subject demonstrates that if the target tumor in this assay displays susceptibility to the new test drug, then the chances of its clinical success are about 80%. However, if the test drug is ineffective in this test, chances of its clinical failure are about 90% for the tested tumor type. Therefore, human tumor cloning assay can provide highly useful information for the ultimate clinical potential of the new agent and help identify tumor types that should receive particular attention.

Thus, with this background information, effects of pMC540 and merodantoin were evaluated against breast cancer and lung (non-small cell) cancer in a human tumor cloning assay.[24-26] These experiments were carried out in collaboration with Dr. Daniel D. Von Hoff, The Cancer Therapy and Research Center, San Antonio, Texas. In these experiments, fresh human breast tumor cells (obtained with informed consent) were suspended in 0.3% agar in enriched CMRL 1066 medium supplemented with 15% heat inactivated horse serum, penicillin (100 units/ml), streptomycin (2 μg/ml), glutamine (2mM), insulin (3 units/ml), asparagine (0.6 mg/ml), Hepes buffer (2 mM). Various doses of pMC540 or merodantoin were then added to the above mixture for continuous drug exposure. The tumor cell containing agar was overlaid on top of an underlayer of agar to prevent the growth of fibroblasts. For each data point three plates were set up and incubated at 37°C. On day 14, plates were removed and colonies consisting of 50 or more cells were counted. The percent surviving fraction was then calculated for each drug dose by comparing it to the number of colonies in control plates. Quality control measures for the determination of evaluable samples, survival of colonies in control plates and positive control agent, orthosodium vanadate, known to destroy all colonogenic cells were employed. A summary of results from these experiments is shown in Table 2.6. For pMC540 83% of the breast and lung tumors were found to be responsive at a dose of 80 μg/ml (140.4 μM). This rate increased to virtually 100% when the dose of pMC540 was increased to 120 μg/ml (210.6 μM). However, the response rate of these tumors to

Table 2.6 Activity of preactivated MC540 and merodantoin in a human tumor cloning assay

Tumor Type	Treatment pMC540 (μg/ml) 80	120	160	Merodantoin (μg/ml) 12.5	25
Breast	4/5	5/5	5/5	0/4	2/4
Lung Carcinoma (non-small cell)	1/1	1/1	1/1	0/1	0/1
Total	5/6	6/6	6/6	0/5	2/5
% response rate	(83)	(100)	(100)	(0)	(40)

** Survival of 50% or less colonies was considered responsive.Doses of pMC540 used: 40 μg/ml (70.2 μM); 80 μg/ml (140.4 μM); 120 μg/ml (210.6 μM); 160 μg/ml (280.8 μM). Doses of merodantoin used: 12.5 μg/ml (51.6 μM); 25 μg/ml (103.3 μM).

merodantoin was only 40% at the highest dose of 25 μg/ml. This low response rate could be explained by the lack of uniform dispersion of merodantoin in aqueous environment due to the hydrophobic nature of this compound. As described in chapter 4, merodantoin was found to be highly effective against solid breast tumor xenografts. Nonetheless, a high degree of susceptibility of patient derived fresh human breast and lung (non-small cell) carcinoma tumors to pMC540 and merodantoin, demonstrates that the chances of their clinical success are very high as dictated by the documented experience with human tumor cloning system.

In Vitro Studies of Viral Inactivation

As stated earlier, the first interaction of a drug with the cell is more likely to be at the plasma membrane. Many properties are expressed at or mediated by the cell surface. It is implicit from much of the published work that viral envelopes bear a close resemblance in terms of overall chemical and physical properties to membranes of host cell from which the virion originates.[27,28] Therefore, we elected to investigate the effects of pMC540 on enveloped viruses. Herpes simplex virus 1 (HSV-1) was the first target because of its availability in our laboratory. These experiments were performed in our virology laboratory in collaboration with Dr. Joseph Newman. Treatment of cell free HSV-1 (Fig. 2.5) with 10 μg/ml (17.55 μM) and 17.5 μg/ml (30.71 μM) of pMC540

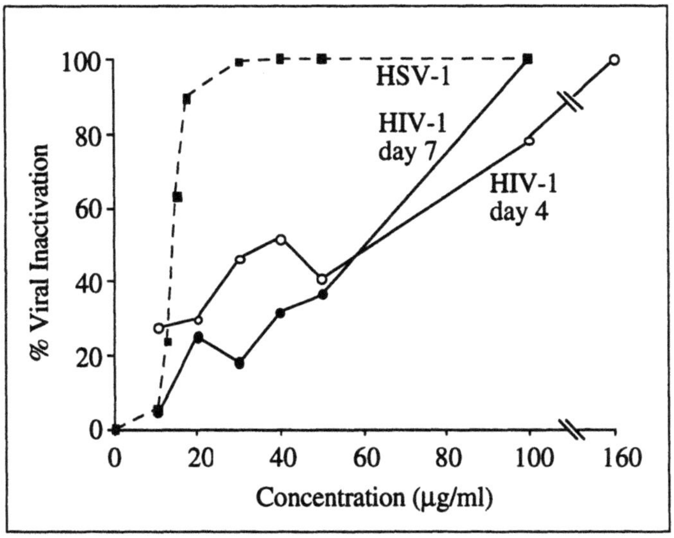

Fig. 2.5 Dose response curves of preactivated merocyanine 540 on herpes simplex virus (HSV-1) and human immunodeficiency virus (HIV-1). Reprinted with permission from: European Journal of Cancer 1990; 26:551-553.

caused a 50% and 90% inactivation of the virus, respectively. Encouraged by these results this study was expanded to include echovirus, adenovirus and human immunodeficiency virus (HIV-1). The non-enveloped echovirus and adenovirus were not affected (Table 2.7) by pMC540 treatment, indicating that the presence of viral envelope was a mandatory condition for the expression of the antiviral activity of this compound.

Subsequent experiments involving immunodeficiency viruses were carried out in collaboration with Dr. Tran Chanh, Department of Virology and Immunology and Center for AIDS Research, Southwest Foundation for Biomedical Research, San Antonio, Texas. A brief period (2 hours) treatment of cell free HIV-1 resulted in a dose dependent inactivation of HIV-1. The 50% and 90% inactivation doses were 60 and 90 μg/ml respectively (Fig. 2.5).

It is interesting to note that another photoactive compound called dihematoporphyrin ether (DHE), a more purified form of HPD, so called at the time and later proved to be a chemically incorrect name, was also preactivated and then used in preliminary experiments of cell free HIV inactivation. Preactivated DHE (50 μg/ml) was also found to be effective in causing over 95% of the HIV inactivation. However, this compound displayed a high degree of non-specific toxicity to normal cells as compared to pMC540 and thus was not pursued any further. Even so, at the

Table 2.7. Effect of preactivated MC540 on the inactivation of non-enveloped adenovirus and echovirus

Conditions	Dose	PFU/ml	% Inactivation	Log Reduction
Control (Ad6)*	0.0 mg/ml	2.8×10^7	–	–
Adenovirus 6	20 mg/ml	2.7×10^7	3.6	0.016
Adenovirus 6	80 mg/ml	2.6×10^7	7.2	0.032
Adenovirus 6	160 mg/ml	2.7×10^7	3.6	0.016
Control (Ech21)*	0.0 mg/ml	1.0×10^5	–	–
Echovirus 21	20 mg/ml	7.5×10^4	25.0	0.12
Echovirus 21	80 mg/ml	9.0×10^4	10.0	0.05
Echovirus 21	160 mg/ml	5.0×10^4	50.0	0.30

Cell free viral suspensions were treated with or without the indicated concentrations of pMC540. After a 20 hour incubation at 37°C, adenovirus and echovirus were assayed in A549 and MRC-5 cells respectively. *Adenovirus type 6 and echovirus type 21. Preactivated MC540 = pMC540. Doses of pMC540 used: 20 µg/ml (35.1 mM); 80 µg/ml (140.4 µM); 160 µg/ml (280.8 µM).

time, its biological activity in the absence of light was a useful observation for us as it provided additional support for the establishment of the fact that 'preactivation' was not limited to a single compound.

Nonetheless, the next step was to determine whether pMC540 was also effective against cell associated HIV-1. To answer this question cultured human T cells (Hut-78) were first infected with HIV-1 and then treated with 200 µg/ml of pMC540. After 2 hours of incubation, the cells were washed to remove the drug and they were resuspended in fresh drug free medium. Viability of cells was evaluated on days 1, 2, 5, 7 and 9. Data from these experiments show that even a brief single dose treatment of HIV-infected human T cells with pMC540 protected over 40% of the treated cells whereas all untreated cells were killed by the virus. These results suggest that pMC540 treatment protects some of the HIV-infected cells by destroying the virus.[29] It is conceivable that prolonged treatment of HIV-infected cells may be significantly more effective in destroying the virus and protecting healthy cells.

It is noteworthy that the main reason for using a high dose but a brief period of treatment was that pMC540 displays preferential cytotoxicity towards activated, transformed, malignant and virus infected cells. Cultured human T cells used in these experiments cannot be considered "normal" cells even if they were originally obtained from healthy individuals. Cultured cells derived from normal donors should never be considered "normal." In the absence of true normal cells, primary cultures of cells derived from normal donors can be considered the closest thing to "normal" cells. There is increasing evidence that the plasma membrane of cultured cells, transformed cells, activated cells and tumor cells differs from that of normal cells. In transformed cells, for example, increased activity to lectins[30] and to anti-glycolipid antibody,[31] incomplete synthesis of carbohydrate chains in glycolipid[32] and glycoproteins,[33] enhanced synthesis of a specific sialylfucopeptide[34] and contact response such as contact inhibition, topoinhibition, contact orientation and contact promotion are particularly notable. The immunologic evidence for antigenic differences between normal and transformed cells[35] and biochemical evidence for changes in surface components upon transformation have been documented.[35] Thus, normal cells placed in culture do not possess properties identical to those of unmanipulated normal cells. Getting back to pMC540, however, the mechanism of this inherent capability of pMC540 to recognize differences in the plasma membranes of malignant, transformed, activated and virus infected cells remains unclear. Nevertheless, this is a highly desirable property. As it will be described in the following chapter, preliminary work is already in progress to enhance our understanding of the structure-activity as it relates to the preferential affinity of pMC540 towards neoplastic cells.

Further studies of the in vitro antiviral activity were designed to determine the extent of viral inactivation achieved by measuring the release of p24 antigen from the living HIV. In these experiments a suspension of cell free HIV-1 was first treated with pMC540 for 2 hours and then used to infect MT-4 cells. In control experiments MT-4 cells were infected with untreated HIV-1. Both control and experimental MT-4 cells thus produced were maintained in cultures and the cell supernatant was analyzed for the amount of p24 antigen released. A two hour treatment of uninfected MT-4 cells treated with either solvent control or pMC540 at doses up to 200 μg/ml (351 μM) did not elicit significant toxicity to these cells. In the control group, the amount of p24 antigen detected on day 4 and 7 were approximately 735 and 956 pg/ml respectively. However, the amount of HIV-1 p24 antigen in MT-4 cultures infected with HIV-1 but treated with pMC540 (80, 160 and 200 μg/ml) was significantly lower, ranging from 7.6 to 9.5 pg/ml on day 4 and 6.8 to 12.4 pg/ml on day 7 of culture. (Table 2.8). Virtually identical results were obtained when simian immunodeficiency virus $(SIV)_{mac251}$ was used. (Table 2.8). Similarly, long-term (21 day) cultures of MT-4 cells infected with pMC540-treated HIV-1 retained a degree of viability comparable to that of control uninfected MT-4 cells. These data demonstrate that a very brief period of treatment with pMC540 was effective in inactivating the cell free HIV-1 and SIV.

Next, in view of the clinical progression of the disease, it was essential to determine whether HIV-infected fresh human peripheral blood mononuclear cells (PBMC) would respond to pMC540 treatment. For this purpose experiments were done in which PHA-activated fresh human PBMC were first infected with HIV-1 for 7 days. The presence of infection was confirmed by virus isolation and then HIV-1 infected cultures were divided into two sets. HIV-infected human PBMC in one set were treated with 351.0 μM pMC540 (200 μg/ml) for 2 hours while the other set was left untreated. Culture supernatants from both sets were collected and analyzed for the amounts of HIV-1 p24 antigens by the antigen-

Table 2.8 Preactivated MC540 inactivates cell-free HIV-1 and SIV

MT-4 Cell Infection		Dose of	Viral Antigens, (pg/ml)*			
			HIV-1		SIV	
HIV-1	SIV	pMC540 (μg/ml)	Day 4	Day 7	Day 4	Day 7
+	–	–	735.3	956.7	–	–
+	–	80.0	9.5	12.4	–	–
+	–	160.0	7.6	6.8	–	–
+	–	200.0	8.1	8.0	–	–
–	+	–	–	–	73.0	65.9
–	+	80.0	–	–	10.4	12.9
–	+	160.0	–	–	4.2	5.0
–	+	200.0	–	–	3.5	2.8

HIV, human immunodeficiency virus; SIV, simian immunodeficiency virus; pMC540, preactivated merocyanine 540. *Mean of duplicate determinations using the antigen-capture enzyme-linked immunosorbent assay kits for HIV and SIV. pMC540 dose: 1 μg/ml = 1.755 μM. Reprinted with permission from Journal of AIDS 1992; 5:188-195.

capture ELISA. Results show that there was a considerable reduction in the amount of p24 antigen in the treated set (Table 2.9). Although these results do not reflect a direct intracellular inactivation of HIV-1 by pMC540, nonetheless, a significant reduction in the amount of p24 antigen released and a concomitant decrease in the percentage of antigen expressing PBMC argues for pMC540 mediated inactivation of HIV-1 infected human PBMC's. This argument is further strengthened by the fact that these results were obtained by a very brief (2 hour) treatment. Longer periods of treatment with very low doses of pMC540 kill the infected cells, thereby destroying the HIV-1 as well as its factory, the virus producing cells. This, after all, is the central goal for any successful treatment of AIDS.

Another important observation made was that treatment of cell free HIV-1 with pMC540 reduced the capacity of HIV-1 to bind to cultured human T cells (Hut-78) as determined by indirect immunofluorescence (Fig. 2.6). However, treatment of target cells instead of HIV-1 with pMC540 did not interfere with HIV-1 or SIV binding. A similar inhibition of HIV-1 binding to normal

Table 2.9. Effect of preactivated MC540 on HIV-1 infected human PBMCs

	Days in culture					
	9		11		15	
Treatment of HIV-1-infected PBMC	p24 (pg/ml)	%*	p24 (pg/ml)	%	p24 (pg/ml)	%
None	10.6	ND	20.0	30.2	49.5	64.4
	12.4		25.1		71.0	
pMC540 (200 μg/ml)	9.2	ND	7.8	4.5	2.2	1.0
	10.7		8.1		2.7	

pMC540, preactivated merocyanine 540; HIV, human immunodeficiency virus; PBMC, human peripheral blood mononuclear cells; ND, not done. Normal human PBMC were infected in vitro with HIV-1 on day 0 of culture. On day 7 postinfection, one aliquot was left untreated while the other was treated with pMC540 for a period of 2 hours at 37° C.
*Antigen-capture enzyme-linked immunosorbent assay (pg/ml) and indirect immunofluorescence assays (percent of PBMC expressing HIV-1 antigens) were done on the days indicated. Reprinted with permission from Journal of AIDS 1992; 5:188-195.

human PBMC was also obtained with pMC540 treatment (Fig. 2.7). This inhibition, however, could not be accounted for by the inability of the anti-HIV-1 serum to bind the treated virions since binding was observed with ELISA assays with treated HIV-1. Nonetheless, these data suggest that pMC540 treatment may be modifying some essential structures on the envelope of the HIV-1, and this structure appears to be different than the one required for anti-HIV-1 serum binding.

The next step was to carry out radioimmunoprecipitation experiments to determine how CD4 binding to gp120 of HIV-1 was affected by treatment with pMC540 (Fig. 2.8). We decided to use a particular murine anti-CD4 mAbs,[36,37] one designated L117, since it binds to a region of CD4 outside the primary gp120

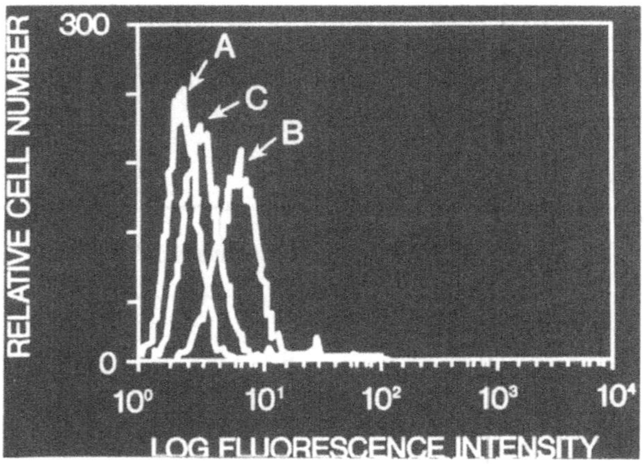

Fig. 2.6. Inhibition of HIV-1 binding to uninfected Hut-78 cells by preactivated merocyanine 540 (pMC540) treatment. Immunofluorescent profiles of Hut-78 cells. (A) Hut-78 + HIV-1+ normal control serum; (B) Hut-78 + HIV-1 + anti-HIV-1 serum; (C) Hut-78 + pMC540 treated HIV-1 + anti-HIV-1 serum. Reprinted with permission from Journal of AIDS 1992; 5:188-195.

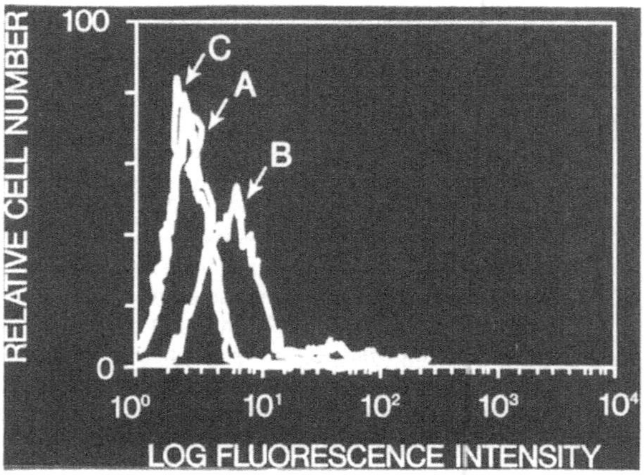

Fig. 2.7. Inhibition of HIV-1 binding to normal human peripheral blood mononuclear cells (PBMC) by pMC540 treatment. (A) PBMC + HIV-1+ normal control serum; (B) PBMC + HIV-1 + anti-HIV-1 serum; (C) PBMC + pMC540 treated HIV-1 + anti-HIV-1 serum. Reprinted with permission from Journal of AIDS 1992; 5:188-195.

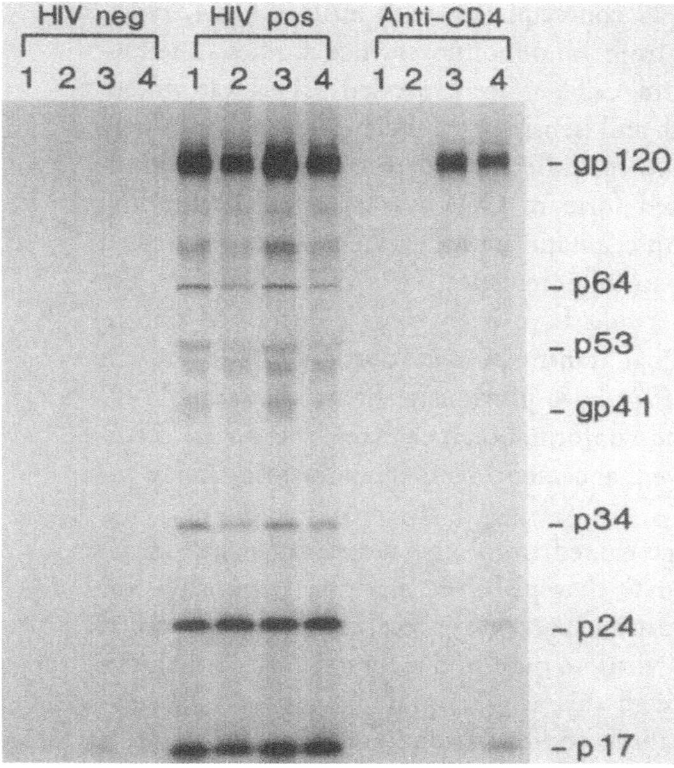

Fig. 2.8. Effects of preactivated merocyanine 540 (pMC540) on human immunodeficiency virus (HIV-1) binding to srCD4. [^{35}S] Cysteine-labeled HIV-1 purified from culture supernatants was subjected to treatment with pMC540 (lanes 2 and 4) or was untreated (lanes 1 and 3) before incubation with srCD4 (lanes 3 and 4) or no srCD4 (lanes 1 and 2). The complexes were then immunoprecipitated with a seronegative human serum, an HIV-1 seropositive human serum, or an anti-CD4 monoclonal antibody (L117). The precipitated proteins were then separated by SDS-polyacrylamide gel electrophoresis followed by autoradiography. Reprinted with permission from Journal of AIDS 1992; 5:188-195.

binding domain, and therefore would be useful for studying CD4 binding to HIV-1 by coprecipitating bound gp120. What we found was a slight reduction in the intensity of gp120, but no effect on the binding to soluble CD4 receptors, nor any significant reduction in either *gag* antigens p24 or p17. These antigens are coprecipitated along with the gp120-srCD4 complex, leading one to speculate that pMC540 is cross-linking the viral membrane. The pMC540 appears to be stabilizing the viral membrane, forming large viral envelope complexes unobservable by radioimmunoprecipitation techniques. Only after solubilizing the membrane in the presence of sodium dodecyl sulfate, reducing with dithiothreitol and boiling the products, were the *gag* antigens partially freed for visualization by gel electrophoresis.

Our radioimmunoprecipitation studies suggest that pMC540 may be mediating its effect some time after receptor binding. In these studies we found no significant differences in soluble CD4 receptor binding in the presence or absence of pMC540, as assessed by the intensity of gp120 coprecipitated with mAb to CD4. However, in data gathered from immunofluorescence studies, a reduction in viral binding to cell surface-expressed CD4 was noted. Differences of method and sensitivity inherent in each of these techniques could account for differences detected in receptor binding. A soluble truncated form of CD4 was used in the binding assays for radioimmunoprecipitation, while cellular CD4 was treated with pMC540 for immunofluorescence. In the latter studies, the conformation of CD4 could have been more constrained due to the additional C-terminal transmembrane portion of the protein missing from srCD4. (We have previously shown that soluble receptors induce profound conformational changes in the viral membrane, associated with enhancement of infection with a simian virus, $SIV_{(agm)}$.[38])

With the knowledge gained from our studies done thus far, it is interesting to speculate that pMC540 may be responsible for viral membrane stabilization, preventing receptor-mediated activation. In order for the virus to fuse and penetrate the cell membrane, it must go through this activation step, induced by receptor binding, which causes conformational rearrangement. It is conceivable that pMC540 treatment inhibits viral conformation changes by stabilizing the viral lipid bilayer membrane, preventing activation and fusion with the cell. Clearly, much more work is required for a better understanding of the mechanism(s) involved in the observed inhibition of HIV binding to its target cell in response to pMC540 treatment.

During the course of this research, upon the suggestion from an official at NIH (during a conversation in 1992 regarding our upcoming grant application and antiviral data), pMC540 was submitted for its evaluation of anti-HIV properties in vitro. The evaluation of antiviral activity and cytotoxicity was performed using CEM human T-lymphocyte cell line. Results from this investigation revealed that pMC540 produced substantial inhibition of viral replication (> 90%) at doses of 100 μg/ml as determined by p24 antigen assay. These results were strikingly similar to what we had previously reported. The same report also revealed that pMC540 was cytotoxic to CEM cells and PHA stimulated normal peripheral blood mononuclear cells as well. In view of the anti-HIV activity, as well as cytotoxicity to cultured cells, pMC540 was considered non-selective leading to the conclusion that further research was not warranted. However, these findings were not new as our very first publication, two years earlier, clearly documented the cytotoxic properties of pMC540 against various cultured cell lines.[18] In this paper, we also demonstrated that pMC540 spares 85% of the true normal (i.e. non-transformed, non-activated, uninfected) cells. We also provided preliminary data from a different laboratory at NIH that treatment of HIV-infected SCID mice with pMC540 (120 mg/kg) given on alternate days provided full protection to 9 out of 10 treated mice.

If pMC540 was really an indiscriminate toxic substance, it should have killed all of the treated animals. However, this was not the case then and has subsequently proven to be correct in the treatment of SIV-infected monkeys, FIV-infected cats and tumor bearing mice as discussed in following chapters. In view of this already known information, we asked for reconsideration of their conclusion without success.

It is important to note that there are serious problems with the conclusions made based upon the NIH in vitro data. 1) If the drug is inactivating the cell free virus and also killing the transformed or activated or infected cells at the same time, it may be non-specific but it is highly desirable for the patient because the main aim is to destroy the virus as well as the virus producing factory, the infected cell. 2) In addition to viral inactivation, if pMC540 also kills the malignant cells (e.g. HIV associated Kaposi's sarcoma), the question should be asked what harm is this going to bring to the patient? As a matter of fact, this is a highly desirable property as it will destroy any susceptible malignancy as well. 3) Cultured normal peripheral mononuclear cells or human T-lymphocyte cell line CEM cells cannot and should not be used as a measure of cytotoxicity to normal cells in lieu of true normal cells because the former are not normal cells as discussed in chapter 1. Clearly, there is an overwhelming need to overcome the erroneous but established paradigm.

In any event, experiments described above demonstrate that laboratory strain of SIV and HIV were quite susceptible to the antiviral activity of pMC540. However, we had no idea whether or not pMC540 would be effective in the inactivation of HIV isolated from a patient. To answer this question, preliminary experiments were set up in which JR-CSF, a low passage, patient-derived HIV isolate was treated with different doses of pMC540.

After overnight incubation at 37 °C, the virus plus pMC540 mixture was added to 1 x 10^6 PHA activated normal peripheral blood mononuclear cells. After 1 hour incubation, the cells were washed and resuspended in 1.0 ml of growth medium. Supernatants from these cultures were harvested on days 3, 6, and 9 for p24 antigen-capture enzyme-linked immuno assays. Results show (Table 2.10) that as little as 17.5 μM (10 μg/ml) of pMC540 was sufficient to cause a virtually complete inactivation of JR-CSF as determined by the undetectable levels of p24. It is noteworthy that viability of uninfected fresh normal human peripheral blood mononuclear cells was 85% when treated with 210.6 μM (120 μg/ml) of pMC540 (12 times the dose that inactivated JR-CSF) for 24 hours. Time kinetics studies revealed that as little as a 2 hour treatment of this virus with 10 μg/ml of pMC540 was sufficient for its virtually complete inactivation as determined by the undetectable levels of p24 antigen. Taken together these data suggest that patient isolate

Table 2.10. Effect of pMC540 on the inactivation of patient derived HIV isolate

Human PBMC	**JR-CSF**	**pMC540** (μg/ml)	**p24 Antigen (pg/ml)** Day 3	Day 6	Day 9
+	–	–	Neg.	Neg.	Neg.
+	+	–	124	244	255
+	+	100	Neg.	Neg.	Neg.
+	+	50	Neg.	Neg.	Neg.
+	+	25	Neg.	Neg.	Neg.
+	+	10	Neg.	Neg.	Neg.
+	+	5	2	178	240
+	+	1	Neg.	100	238

Patient derived HIV isolate JR-CSF was treated with different doses of pMC540. After overnight incubation at 37 °C, virus dye mixture was added to 1 x 10^6 PHA activated human peripheral blood mononuclear cells. After 1 hour of incubation, cells were washed and resuspended in 1.0 ml of fresh growth medium. Supernatants were collected on day 3, 6 and 9 for p24 antigen-capture analysis by ELISA. Mean values of a duplicate determination are shown. pMC540 dose: 1 mg/ml = 1.755 mM. pMC540 = preactivated merocyanine 540; JR-CSF = low passage, patient-derived HIV isolate; PBMC = human peripheral blood mononuclear cells; Neg. = p24 undetectable

JR-CSF strain of HIV is more sensitive to the virucidal activity of pMC540 than the laboratory strain.

Thus, in conclusion, preactivated merocyanine 540 was found to be very effective as an anticancer and antiviral agent in vitro. At the same time this agent spared the majority of normal cells, a much sought after property in any chemotherapeutic agent. The fact that pMC540 is effective against virus as well as tumor cells raises one apparently irreconcilable question from the mechanistic point of view, i.e. how can an agent attack two completely diverse targets? However, the question is not irreconcilable at all when one considers the fact that viral envelopes bear a close resemblance to membrane of the host cell from which the virion originates.[28,29] During the course of its replication cycles, the virion could have originated from a diverse type of cells eventually acquiring many properties of the plasma cell membrane while preserving its own. In this context, it is perhaps important to reiterate that pMC540 was found to be totally ineffective against non-enveloped viruses such as echovirus or adenovirus, suggesting that the antitumor and antiviral activity of pMC540 must be dependent upon some initial interaction with the component(s) of the plasma membranes, an area wide open for further research.

References

1. Sogandares-Bernal F, Matthews JL, Judy MM. HPD-induced reversal of chloroquine resistance of malaria. Mem Inst Oswaldo Cruz, Rio de Janeiro, 1986; 81:241-50.
2. Salama G, and Murad M. Merocyanine 540 as an optical probe of transmembrane electrical activity in the heart. Science 1976; 191:485-87.
3. Atzpodien J, Gulati SC, Clarkson BD. Comparison of cytotoxic effects of merocyanine 540 on leukemic cells and human bone marrow. Cancer Res 1986; 46:4892- 94.
4. Sieber F. Marrow purging by merocyanine 540 mediated photolysis. Bone Marrow Transplantation. Proceedings of the First International Workshop on Bone Marrow Purging 1987; 2:(Suppl. 2)29-33.
5. Gulliya KS, Pervaiz S. Elimination of clonogenic tumor stem cells from HL-60, Daudi and U-937 cell lines by laser photoradiation therapy: Implication for A bone marrow purging. Blood 1989; 73:1059-1065.
6. Gulliya K, Fay J, Dowben R et al. Elimination of leukemic cells by photodynamic therapy. Cancer Chemother Pharmacol 1988; 22:211-14.

7. Gulliya K, Matthews J, Fay J et al. Increased survival of bone marrow cells during laser light induced photosensitization: Implications for ex vivo bone marrow purging. Life Sci 1988; 112: 2651-56.
8. Gulliya KS. An in vitro model of autologous bone marrow purging for multiple myeloma and lung carcinoma cells by laser photoradiation therapy. Cancer J 1989; 2:378-82.
9. Gulliya KS, Battaglino M. Breast cancer and laser photoradiation therapy: An in vitro model of autologous bone marrow purging. In: Gross S, Gee AP, Worthington-White DA, eds. Prog Clin Biol Res. New York: Wiley-Liss, 1989: 133:103-107.
10. Chan WS, Sevenson R, Phillips D et al. Cell uptake, distribution and response to aluminumchloro sulfonated phthalocyanine: a potential antitumor photosensitizer. Br J Cancer 1986; 53:255-63.
11. van Lier JE, Spikes JD. The chemistry, photophysics and photosensitizing properties of of phthalocyanines. In: Bock G, Harnett Wiley S, eds. Photosensitizing Compounds: Their Chemistry, Biology and Clinical Use. Chichester: Ciba Foundation, 1989: 146:17-26.
12. Rosenthal I, Murali Krishna C, Risez P et al. The role of molecular oxygen in the photodynamic effect of phthalocyanines. Radiat Res 1986; 107:136-42.
13. Weishaupt KR, Gomer CJ, Dougherty TJ. Identification of singlet oxygen as the cytotoxic agent in the inactivation of a murine tumor. Cancer Res 1976; 36:2326-29.
14. Moan J. On the diffusion length of singlet oxygen in cells and tissues. J Photochem Photobiol B Biol 1990, 6:343-44.
15. Davila J, Harriman A, Gulliya KS et al. Photochemistry of merocyanine 540: The mechanism of chemotherapeutic activity with cyanine dyes. Photochem Photobiol 1991; 53:1-11.
16. Longo DL. Lung Cancer: The (red) light at the end of tunnel? Abstract and commentary. Clinical Oncology Alert 1993; 8:91-92.
17. Chang Po-H, Pervaiz S, Battaglino M et al. Synergistic effect of preactivated photofrin-II and tamoxifen in killing retrofibroma pseudomyxoma and breast cancer cells. Eur J Cancer 1991; 28:1034-39.
18. Gulliya KS, Pervaiz S, Dowben et al. Tumor cell specific dark cytotoxicity of light-exposed merocyanine 540: Implications for systemic therapy without light. Photochem Photobiol 1990; 51:831-38.
19. Singh RJ, Feix JB, Kalyanaraman B. Photobleaching of merocyanine 540: involvement of singlet molecular oxygen. Photochem Photobiol 1992; 55:483-89.
20. Spikes JD. Quantum yields and kinetics of the photobleaching of hematoporphyrin, photofrin II, tetra (4-sulfonatophenyl)-porphine and uroporphyrin. Photochem Photobiol 1992; 55:797-808.
21. Castell JV, Gomez-Lechon MJ, Grassa C et al. Involvement of drug-derived peroxides in the phototoxicity of naproxen and tiaprofenic acid. Photochem Photobiol 1993; 57:486-90.

22. Ashwood-Smith MJ, Ceska O, Warrington PJ et al.The photobiological activity of 5-geranoxypsoralen and its photoproducts. Photochem Photobiol 1992; 55:529-32.
23. Franck B, Schneider U. Photooxidation products of merocyanine 540 formed under preactivation conditions for tumor therapy. Photochem Photobiol 1992; 56:271-76.
24. Hamburger AW, Salmon SE. Primary bioassay of human tumor stem cells. Science 1977; 197:461-63.
25. Salmon SE, Hamburger AW, Soehnlen B et al. Quantitation of differential sensitivity of human tumor stem cells to anticancer drugs. N Eng J Med 1978; 298:1312-27.
26. Shoemaker RH, Wolpert-Defillipes MK, Kern DH et. al. Application of a human tumor colony-forming assay to new drug screening. Cancer Res 1985; 45:2145-53.
27. Blough HA, Tiffany JM, eds. Cell Membranes and Viral Envelopes. New York: Academic Press, 1980; 2:459-518.
28. Barnhart ER, Ash RJ. Similarities and differences between viral and cellular membranes. Prog Med Virol 1979; 25:89-112.
29. Chanh TC, Allan JS, Pervaiz S. Preactivated merocyanine 540 inactivates HIV-1 and SIV: Potential therapeutic and blood banking applications. J AIDS 1992; 5:188-95.
30. Inbar M, Sachs L. Interaction of the carbohydrate-binding protein concanavalin A with normal and transformed cells. Proc Nat Acad Sci USA 1969; 63:1418-25.
31. Hakamori S, Teather C, Andrews HD. Biochem Biophys Res Commun 1968; 33.563-68.
32. Hakomori S, Teather C, Andrews HD. Glycolipids of hamster fibroblasts and derived malignant-transformed cell lines. Proc Natl Acad Sci USA 1968; 59:254-261.
33. Critchley DR, Macpherson I. Cell density dependent glycolipids in NILz hamster cells. Biochem Biophys Acta 1973; 296:145-59.
34. Grimes WJ. Glycosyltransferase and sialic acid levels of normal and transformed cells. Biochemistry 1973; 12:990-96.
35. Warren L, Fuhrer JB, Buck CA. Surface glycoproteins of normal and transformed cells: a difference determined by sialic acid and a growth-dependent sialyl transferase. Proc Nat Acad Sci USA 1972; 69:1838-42.
36. Klein G. Tumor-specific transplantation antigens: G. H. A Clowes memorial lecture (Review).Cancer Res 1968; 28:625-35.
37. Allan JS, Strauss J, Buck DW. Enhancement of SIV infection with soluble receptor molecules. Science 1990; 247:1084-88.
38. Moore JP, McKeating JA, Weiss, RA. Dissociation of gp 120 from HIV-1 virions induced by soluble CD4. Science 1990; 250:1139-42.

CHAPTER 3

PHOTOCHEMISTRY AND PHOTOPHYSICS OF MEROCYANINE 540

Anthony A. Harriman

Every great advance in science has issued from a new audacity of imagination. —John Dewey (1859-1952) The Quest for Certainty, Ch. II

BACKGROUND

The instrumentation at the Center for Fast Kinetics Research was intended to monitor very fast processes, such as time-resolved fluorescence or pulse radiolysis, in an effort to identify important but highly reactive intermediates. Knowing the nature and fate of these intermediates is of great value for formulating reaction mechanisms and, once the mechanism is known, optimizing the process of interest. A few days spent with such equipment generates a great wealth of experimental data, often requiring a month or more to analyze and decipher. In three days, it is certainly possible to uncover many facets of a chemical or biochemical process. However, deep investigation into complex reaction mechanisms demands regular bursts of experimentation. Such equipment is extremely expensive, requiring constant attention by specialists, and can be difficult to operate properly. More often than not, more than one instrument is needed to tackle a particular research project. Data analysis brings additional difficulties and misinterpretations are common.

Novel Chemotherapeutic Agents: Preactivation in the Treatment of Cancer and AIDS, by K. S. Gulliya.

One solution to this problem is to concentrate the equipment in a regional or national center that researchers can visit for a brief period and conduct their experiments. This principle, which is highly cost-effective, brings with it a continual headache for the director of any such resource: namely, who decides which projects will be studied at the center? There is no satisfactory solution to this question and the NIH changes its guidelines and priorities at an alarming frequency. The biggest obstacle always raised at review boards is that a researcher can have a grant application rejected by the NIH, but can still perform research on that project at an NIH supported facility. Antoher major difficulty was that approximately 90% of the current projects of this NIH supported facility belonged in the category of dubious biomedical relevance and less than 5% of all users held an NIH grant. Thus, urgent action was needed to redress the balance by allowing more projects with biomedical applications in compliance with the NIH guidelines.

THE FIRST ENCOUNTER

Kirpal Gulliya from the Baylor Research Foundation (now Baylor Research Institute) in Dallas, arrived at the Center for Fast Kinetics Research in Austin and began to inquire as to how best to proceed with his investigations. I learned that he was an immunologist and cell biologist but had no prior knowledge of transient spectroscopy, only the basic understanding of photochemistry, little if any comprehension of fast kinetics related computing and an abhorrence of physical chemistry. Within the limits set by the secrecy that seems to be inherent to all biomedical researchers, we set to work. It turned out that our objective was to determine the photophysical properties of a pink dye that was dissolved in aqueous ethanol. The identity of the dye was not to be disclosed but I was assured that the material showed great potential as a means of treating leukemic cells. As it turned out, the project lasted about five years, resulting in a series of publications and presentations at international conferences and several patents.

I volunteered to perform the necessary experiments along with Dr. Gulliya. We quickly found evidence that the dye formed a reasonably long-lived triplet excited state. Furthermore, we were able to demonstrate that this triplet reacted with dissolved oxygen to produce singlet molecular oxygen, albeit in very low quantum yield. My scant knowledge about matters relating to photodynamic therapy was sufficient for me to recall that the most popular reason offered by the scientific community to explain the occurrence of light-induced cytotoxicity involved in situ generation of singlet molecular oxygen.

In time, Dr. Gulliya admitted that the dye was a commercially-available merocyanine dye. It was a piece of straightforward detective work for me to recognize it as being merocyanine 540. I promised to compute the various parameters that had been measured and to send them to Dallas, together with hard copy of all the spectra and an explanation of their meaning, over the weekend.

THE FINAL BOMBSHELL OF THE DAY

Before he returned to Dallas, Dr. Gulliya mentioned, "We have evidence that the reactive intermediate has a lifetime of several days, even a few months if we store the solution, after illumination, in a freezer." We had just established the triplet lifetime as being somewhat less than a millisecond while singlet molecular oxygen survived for about 10 microseconds under the experimental conditions used. He continued, "In our experiments we illuminate the solution overnight, before mixing it with a suspension of the cells. I call this approach 'preactivation' since the photonic energy is stored in the molecule before it penetrates into the cell. In this way, it differs from conventional photodynamic therapy, where it is necessary to illuminate the dye after it has assimilated into the cell."

The next week Dr. Gulliya requested a second visit to Austin in order to complete the investigation and to discuss how to identify this mysterious long-lived intermediate. In time for the next visit, I had arranged for a literature survey covering the known photophysics of merocyanine 540. It appeared that quite a lot was already known about this dye. We agreed that I would complete our preliminary studies with the intention of writing a joint publication describing the photophysical properties of the dye in alcoholic solutions. My interest was aroused by our tentative finding that the quantum yield for formation of the triplet excited state was extremely low, an observation that seemed consistent with the (nonquantitative) literature reports, and that the yield of singlet molecular oxygen was barely detectable. How could a dye be a very effective photosensitizer for killing biological cells if the triplet state was formed in such appallingly low yield? This point was worthy of further consideration and was something that could be investigated with our unique arsenal of sophisticated instruments. The notion of 'preactivation' was pushed to the back of my mind, although I was never allowed to forget it completely, whilst we studied the fundamental question regarding what happens upon illumination of merocyanine 540 in fluid solution.

With the aid of a very capable postdoctoral associate, the photophysical properties of merocyanine 540 soon became apparent. Excitation of the dye in ethanol solution resulted in fluorescence (15%), intersystem-crossing to the triplet manifold (1%), and internal conversion (84%). The latter process involved isomerization of the central double bond and an unstable photoisomer was formed in very high yield. This species returned to the original structure on the time scale of a few milliseconds, in the dark, but was itself extremely photoactive. Isomerization involves frictional forces with the surrounding solvent molecules such that the rate decreases markedly with increasing viscosity of the solvent or with decreasing temperature. It was further shown that excitation produces a change in polarity of the molecule and, therefore, the magnitude of its interaction with adjacent solvent molecules. This means that it is essentially impossible to predict what might be the photophysical properties of the dye after assimilation into a leukemic cell. In any case, the dye was poorly soluble in water and formed a variety of aggregates. It later became possible to measure the photophysical properties of merocyanine 540 dispersed inside leukemic cells. We were able to fully describe the photophysics of the dye and to speculate on its possible modes for achieving light-induced cytotoxicity.

Our main contention was that the ineffective population of the triplet state, which never exceeded 1%, was inconsistent with the dye being a good sensitizer for production of singlet molecular oxygen. On this basis, we surmised that light-induced cytotoxicity did not arise solely from production of singlet molecular oxygen that, in turn, attacked vital cell functions and/or destroyed membranes. We raised the possibility that the photoisomer was somehow involved in cytotoxicity, heat deposited in the system by way of rapid internal conversion could contribute towards cytotoxicity and in situ bleaching of the dye resulted in formation of a cytotoxic product. The latter possibility, which was clearly demonstrated by experiment, was the closest we could come to finding a 'stable' intermediate. It should be remembered, however, that our facilities were expressly designed to study highly reactive species and not to identify products. On this basis, we had gone as far as we could go with the project and it was time to move on. The following chapters illustrate our attempts to understand exactly why merocyanine 540 exerts such a potent cytotoxic effect towards malignant cells.

With direct financial support from the NIH, we began the process of synthesizing derivatives of merocyanine 540 that might help us address the question of mechanism and improve the performance of the dye. At least in the latter quest, if not the former, we were spectacularly successful. It was during this period, however, that I realized for the first time, that killing cancer cells was but only a small part of the overall requirement for effective therapy. Attention had to be given to designing a proper system that preferentially recognizes leukemic cells. Some of our synthetic analogs allowed us to tackle this daunting task, as described in detail late in this chapter, and this is, in my opinion, one of the most valuable parts of our work. What we achieved during this project was only made possible by our ability to both synthesize new derivatives and to conduct a detailed spectroscopic evaluation of their properties.

But what of preactivation? Whilst I accepted the challenge to find the elusive mechanism for light-induced cytotoxicity and structural properties that play an important role in the recognition of malignant cells, Dr. Gulliya persisted in his claims that a long-lived intermediate was the primary reactive species. We tried unsuccessfully to isolate this species. However, Dr. Buchard Franck, University of Münster, Germany, successfully isolated and characterized three photoproducts from preactivated merocyanine 540. Later, we were able to synthesize merodantoin, one of the most potent of these photoproducts, in 50 gram quantities for the majority of in vivo data collected thus far. Biological data obtained by using these isolated compounds appears in following chapters. Finally, I believe that we resolved the issue, removing the barriers to a full understanding of the concept, and rationalized all of our separate findings.

The above narrative is an account of how I became involved in preactivation and, in fact, in the general field of photodynamic therapy. In studying the photophysical properties of merocyanine 540 we tried to stick to the fundamental issues, especially the mechanics of isomerization, and not worry about its biological properties. We had characterized the dye and its precursors by high-resolution mass spectrometry, proton and carbon-13 nuclear magnetic resonance, infrared spectroscopy and elemental composition. In this chapter we present a general description of our work and its apparent significance. As in all areas of science, time is the true test of validity. Let us, therefore, consider some alternatives with an open mind.

UNDERSTANDING THE PHOTOREACTIONS OF MEROCYANINE 540

GROUND-STATE STRUCTURE

Merocyanine 540 (MC540) was developed originally as a dye for the sensitization of photographic plates toward visible light;[1] as its name implies, the principle absorption maximum is located around 540 nm when the dye is adsorbed onto the surface of a colloidal particle. The molecular structure of the dye can be considered to consist of five major components (Fig. 3.1). These components refer to the benzoxazole subunit which functions as an electron donor, the water-solubilizing propylsulfonate chain, the polyene bridge which provides the main structural attribute, the thiobarbiturate subunit which acts as an electron acceptor and the

Fig. 3.1. Structure of MC540.

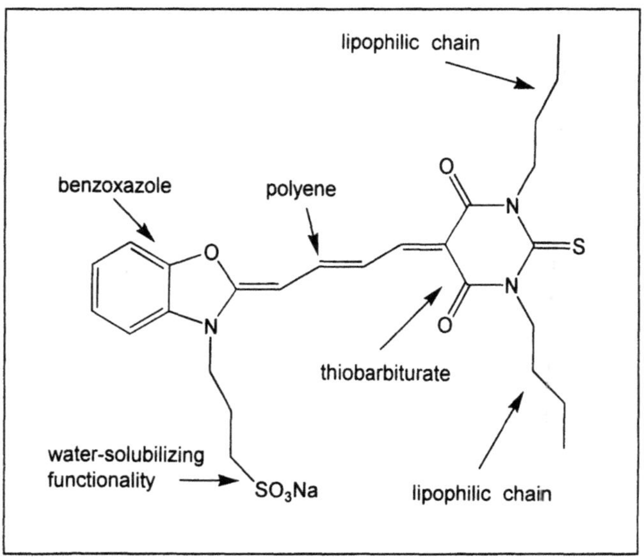

butyl chains that provide increased lipophilicity. Each of these structural units can be modified by straightforward synthetic procedures, thereby generating a wide range of derivatives, such that, in particular, the lipophilicity can be fine-tuned. The dye can be synthesized in large quantities by a long series of simple steps, as illustrated in Figure 3.2. The overall synthesis requires preparation of a suitably alkylated thiobarbituric acid derivative which can be fitted with an alkene chain upon treatment with 1,3,3-trimethoxy-

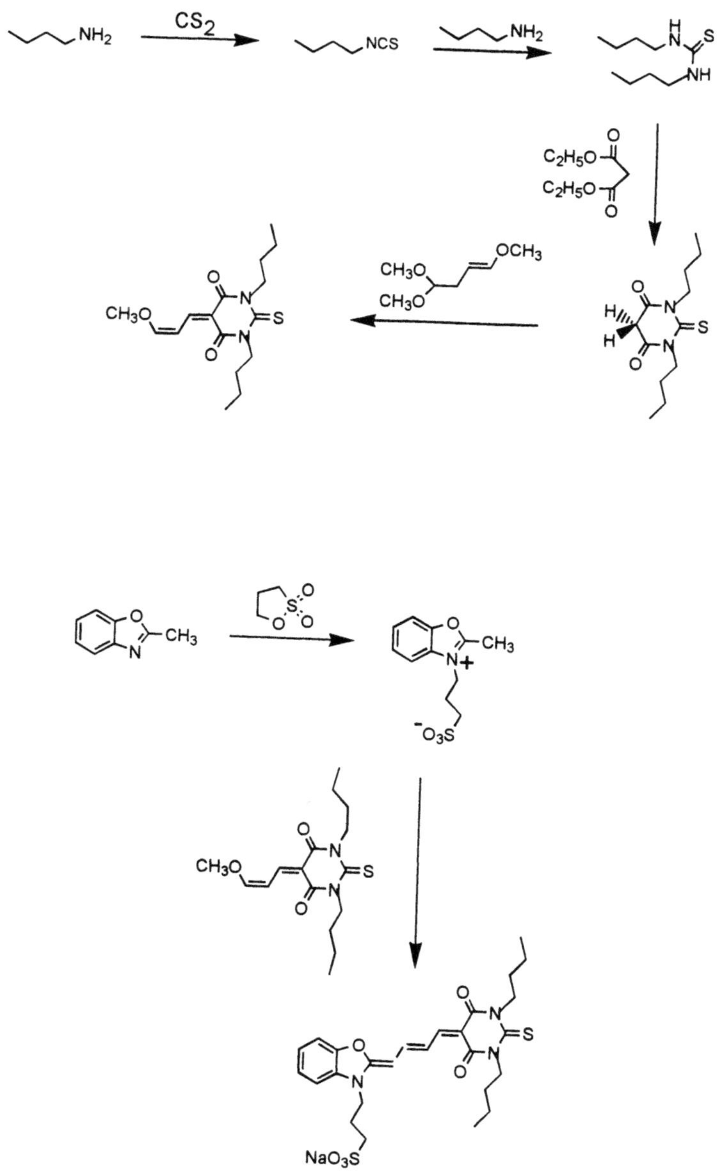

Fig. 3.2. Synthetic scheme used to prepare MC540 from readily available reagents.

propen-1-ene. Subsequent coupling between this latter reagent and the benzoxazole precursor affords the desired merocyanine dye in moderate yield. Purification requires extensive solvent extraction to remove adsorbed amine, recrystallization from ethyl acetate/hexane mixtures and chromatography on silica in order to produce analytically pure material. According to this synthetic methodology, it is convenient to isolate the dye as the triethylammonium salt. If required, this cation, which tends to be hydroscopic and unsuitable for long-term storage, is readily exchanged for sodium by ion-exchange chromatography.

Early attempts to determine the structure of MC540 in solution relied upon resonance Raman spectroscopy,[2] but were not entirely successful because of artifacts introduced by the intense fluorescence emanating from the dye. Similarly, molecular mechanics calculations, which indicated an all *trans* arrangement of the polymethine bridge,[2] were not fully convincing. Instead, we turned to high resolution nuclear magnetic resonance (NMR) spectroscopy[3] to solve the solution-phase structure of the water-insoluble derivative **1** (Structure 3.1). Thus, high field (500 MHz) ^1H NMR COSY spectra were recorded for merocyanine **1** in $CDCl_3$ and are shown in Figures. 3.3 and 3.4. Complete assignment of all the protons in the molecule was possible and the derived chemical shifts and coupling constants are collected in Table 3.1. In particular, the alkenic protons could be clearly identified and assigned. Thus, H(9) was unambiguously identified from its characteristic chemical shift (δ = 5.59) and doublet pattern. For this proton, the measured coupling constant (J) was found to be 12.5 Hz. Three other

*Structure 3.1. Structure of the water-insoluble merocyanine dye **1**.*

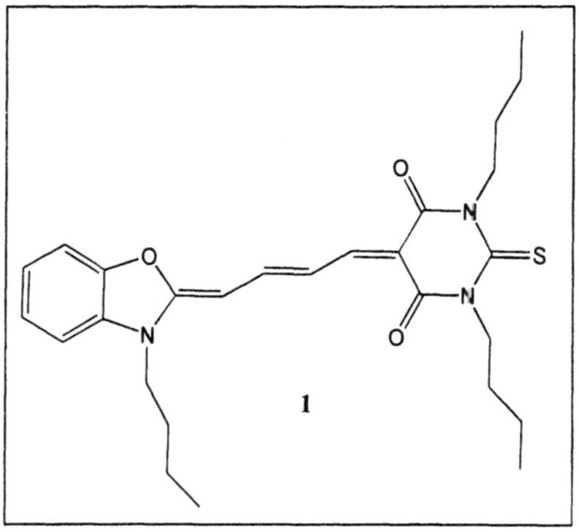

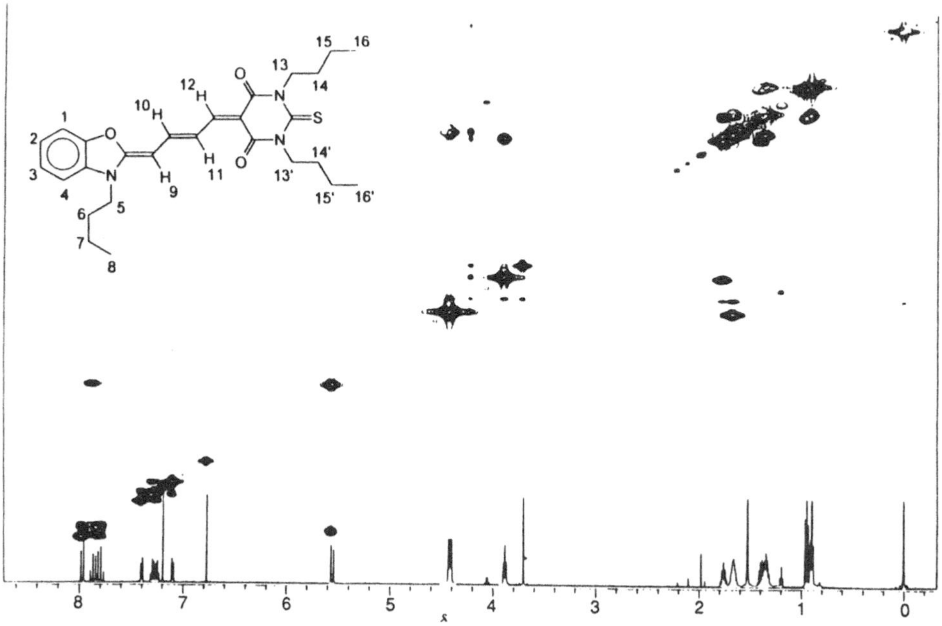

*Fig. 3.3. High-resolution (500 MHz) two-dimensional COSY NMR spectrum recorded for merocyanine **1** in $CDCl_3$, showing the atom labeling. Reprinted with permission from J Chem Soc Faraday Trans 1994; 90:953-961.*

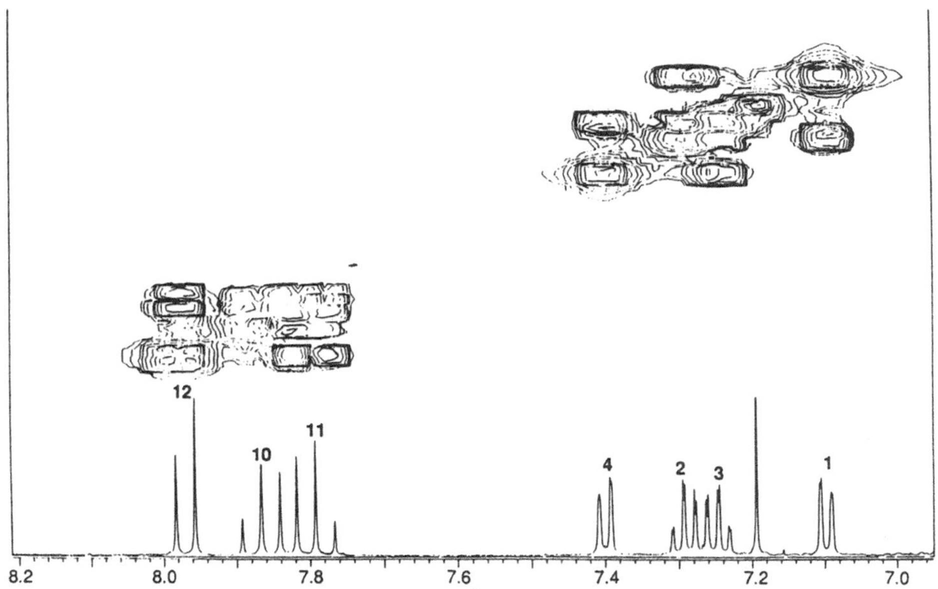

*Fig. 3.4. The (500 MHz) two-dimensional COSY NMR spectrum recorded for merocyanine **1** in $CDCl_3$ showing the expanded aromatic and alkenic regions. Reprinted with permission from J Chem Soc Faraday Trans 1994; 90:953-961.*

Table 3.1. ***^1H NMR spectral properties recorded for merocyanine 1 in $CDCl_3$ solution (see ref. 3)***

Atom Label	Proton Shift,[a] δ	Coupling Constant,[b] J/Hz
16, 16'	0.88-0.91	7.3, 2.0
8	0.91-0.96	7.3
15, 15'	1.31-1.35	c
7	1.36-1.41	c
14, 14'	1.62-1.68	c
6	1.72-1.78	c
5	3.86-3.89	7.3
13, 13'	4.39-4.42	7.8
9	5.54-5.64	12.5
1	7.09-7.11	7.7
3	7.23-7.26	7.8, 1.0
2	7.28-7.31	7.7, 1.2
4	7.39-7.41	8.0
11	7.77-7.82	13.0
10	7.84-7.89	12.9
12	7.95-7.98	13.0

(a) ± 0.1 ppm referenced to TMS; (b) ± 0.1 Hz; (c) too much resonance overlap to evaluate coupling constant.

resonances were observed to possess very similar J values; δ = 7.80 (J = 13.0 Hz), δ = 7.87 (J = 12.9 Hz) and δ = 7.96 (J = 13.0 Hz). These latter three resonances are assignable, therefore, to the remaining three alkenic protons; the observed patterns of two triplets and a doublet being consistent with this assertion. Individual peak assignments could be made from the two-dimensional NMR spectra which indicated mutual coupling between adjacent protons. The second doublet (δ = 7.96) was clearly due to H(12) while the two triplets were assignable to H(10) (δ = 7.87) and H(11) (δ = 7.80). Since the coupling constants found for the alkenic protons were essentially the same, we can conclude that a single type of double bond prevails. On this basis, the ground state conformation must be either all *trans* or all *cis*. Furthermore, since an all *cis* arrangement cannot be accommodated for merocyanine **1**, we conclude that the only acceptable ground state conformation is all *trans*. Detailed analysis of all the resonances indicated that only this single isomer was present to the observable limit (> 95%).

The average magnitude of the coupling constant for the alkenic protons (J = 12.9 Hz) is significantly lower than the value anticipated[4] for an isolated *trans* double bond (J ≈ 17 Hz); the corresponding value for an isolated *cis* double bond is about 10 Hz. This finding is consistent with each of the carbon atoms in the polymethine bridge possessing partial double bond character, as expected for a merocyanine dye which can exist in zwitterionic resonance forms (Structure 3.2). Indeed, the coupling constants for individual protons are seen to increase as that proton nears the thiobarbiturate subunit, owing to an increased electron density.[3] This effect can be interpreted in terms of zwitterionic structures formed by electron donation from the N atom in the benzoxazole subunit to one of the carbonyl groups in the thiobarbiturate subunit.

In the all *trans* conformation, the carbonyl groups on the thiobarbiturate subunit are coplanar with the polymethine bridge and are well positioned for intramolecular hydrogen bonding. Indeed, Fourier transform infra-red (FTIR) spectra indicate the existence of such hydrogen bonding in the solid state (Structure 3.3), as evidenced by a broad absorption band centered at 3400 cm^{-1}. The

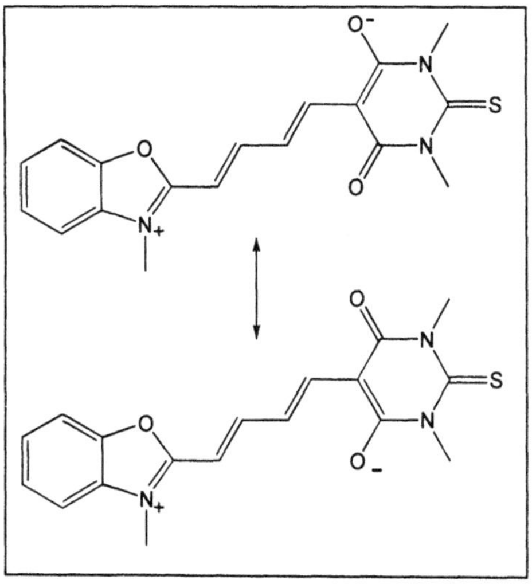

Structure 3.2. Some structures of the zwitterionic form of MC540.

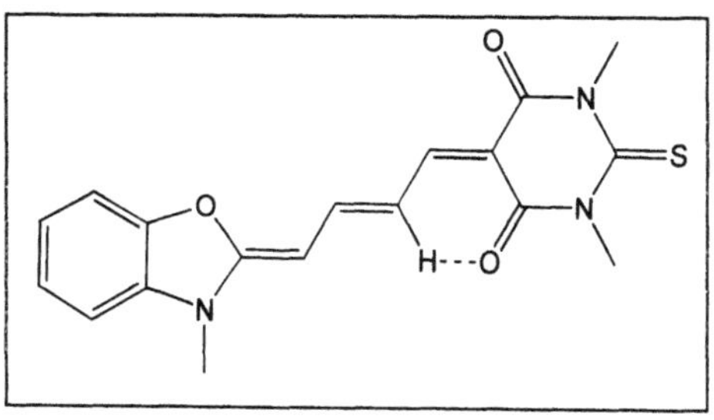

Structure 3.3. Hydrogen bonding observed in the solid state.

carbonyl groups appear[3] as a broad peak centered at 1630 cm^{-1} and a somewhat less intense and sharper peak centered at 1670 cm^{-1}. For a vinylogous amide carbonyl group in the absence of hydrogen bonding, we would expect to observe the CO stretching band at 1670 cm^{-1}. Hydrogen bonding, of medium strength, is expected to lower this frequency by about 30 cm^{-1}. On this basis, the carbonyl band centered at 1670 cm^{-1} is assigned to a non-hydrogen bonded group and the corresponding peak centered at 1630 cm^{-1} is attributed to the hydrogen bonded counterpart.

The presence of zwitterionic resonance forms is also apparent from the measured dipole moment. Thus, merocyanine **1** was found to possess a dipole moment of 10.2 D, making the compound relatively polar. To a considerable approximation, we can consider that the observed dipole moment (μ_{obs}) is a linear combination of dipole moments for the nonpolar form (μ_{np}) and for the fully ionized form (μ_{ion}).[5]

$$(\mu_{obs}) = \alpha(\mu_{np}) + \beta(\mu_{ion}) \qquad (1)$$

Here, the coefficients α and β refer to the fraction of that particular resonance form that contributes to the overall structure. The non-zwitterionic form is expected to exhibit a dipole moment (μ_{np}) of only about 3 D whereas the fully ionized form would be highly polar, the dipole moment (μ_{ion}) being estimated to be about 48 D on the basis of computer calculated molecular dimensions (Structure 3.4). Taking these latter estimates as being absolute values, we conclude that the ground state structure consists predominantly of the nonpolar form ($\alpha \approx 84\%$) but with a sizable ($\beta \approx 16\%$) contribution from the polar form.

Structure 3.4. Dimensions of MC540.

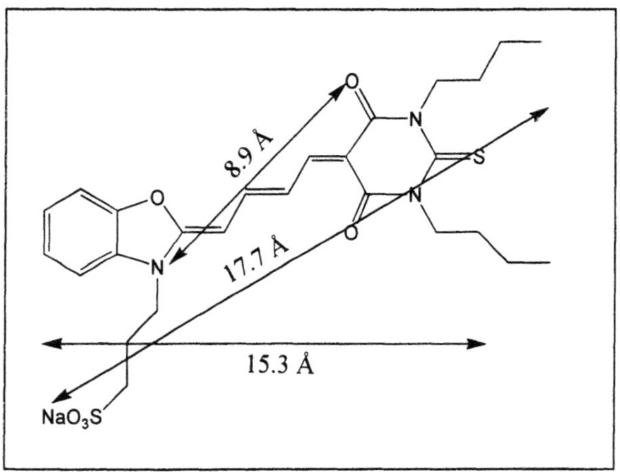

What this means is that the alternating single bonds in the polymethine bridge must possess some degree of double bond character and that, because of the presence of polar resonance structures, there will be preferential alignment of polar solvent molecules around the dye. In other words, polar solvents will tend to stabilize the zwitterionic forms. It is important to bear this point in mind when considering the structure of the dye in a lipid membrane and also when speculating on how the environment might influence the photophysical properties of such merocyanine dyes. As we will see later, the photophysical properties are extremely sensitive to the nature of the surrounding medium.

When considering possible zwitterionic resonance forms that the dye might adapt, it is pertinent to recall that a simple amide can exhibit polar structures that restrict rotation about the C-N bond (Structure 3.5). In respect to merocyanine dyes, this has the effect of extending the conjugation pathway to include the thiobarbiturate subunit, especially the terminal sulfur atom. In this way, conjugation should be considered to run along the entire molecular backbone, resulting in a rigid configuration.

Because of this coexistence of polar and nonpolar forms, MC540 is poorly soluble in both water and alkane solvents. In aqueous media, the dye is present in a highly aggregated form, as evidenced by its absorption spectrum. Addition of a protein, such as human low density lipoprotein (LDL) or a polar organic solvent, such as ethanol, causes monomerization of the dye aggregate (Fig. 3.5). In the case of LDL, the dye is bound to the protein surface,[6] presumably by way of electrostatic interactions, although the rate of uptake is very slow. It appears that about 10-12 dye molecules can be accommodated on a single molecule of LDL (Fig. 3.6), the latter macromolecule having a molecular weight of about 770,000 Daltons, without disrupting the structure or function of the protein. Unlike the situation in pure water, the bound

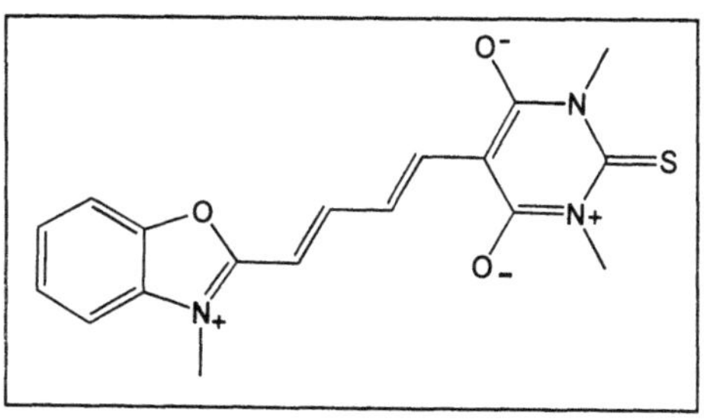

Structure 3.5. Extended conjugation possible for MC540.

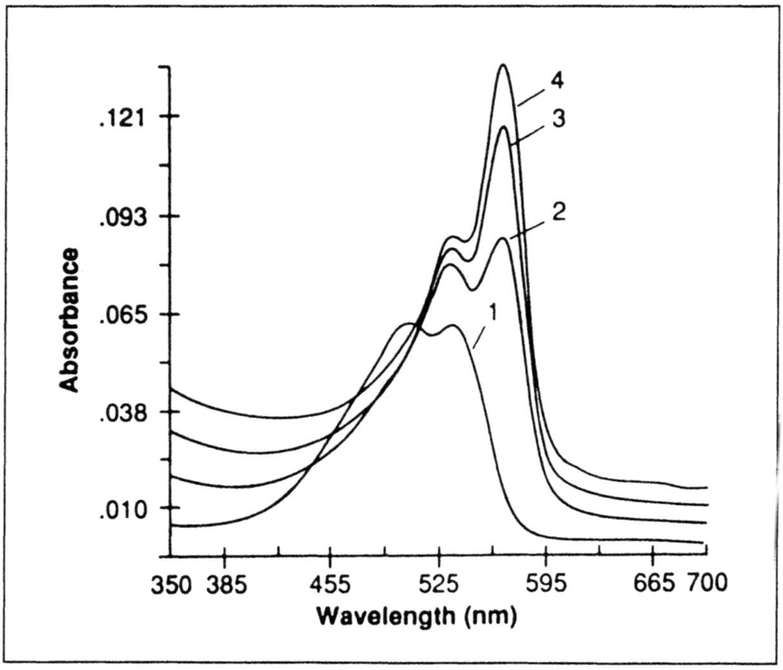

Fig. 3.5. Absorption spectral changes observed upon adding LDL to an aqueous solution of MC540: (1) [MC540] = 1.81 μM, without LDL, (2) [MC540] = 1.76 μM, [LDL] = 0.20 μM, (3) [MC540] = 1.71 μM, [LDL] = 0.40 μM, (4) [MC540] = 1.67 μM, [LDL] = 0.58 μM. Reprinted with permission from The Cancer Journal 1990; 3:360-365.

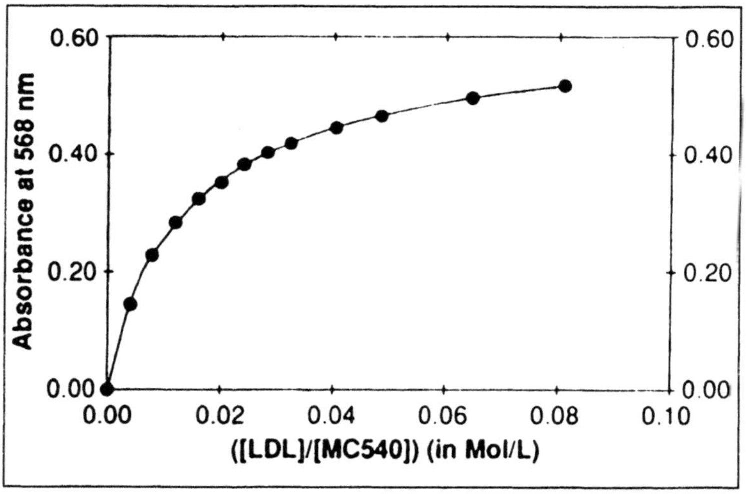

Fig. 3.6. Progressive increase in absorbance characteristic of LDL-bound MC540 (measured at 568 nm) as the molar ratio of LDL to MC540 is increased. The absorbance values were corrected for minor changes in solution volume and for any light scattering arising from the LDL. Reprinted with permission from The Cancer Journal 1990; 3:360-365.

dye is highly fluorescent (Fig. 3.7). This suggests that the dye is bound in a relatively hydrophobic and rigid location on the protein, where it is screened from the surrounding solvent.

At higher dye concentrations, there is an additional uptake of merocyanine dye onto the protein such that a total of about 50 dye molecules can be bound to a single protein molecule (Fig. 3.8.).

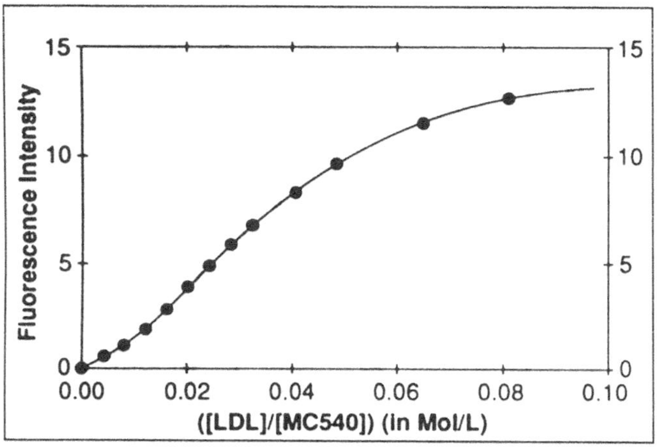

Fig. 3.7. Increase in total fluorescence intensity (excitation at 550 nm) as the molar ratio of LDL to MC540 increases. These data points correspond to the absorption spectral results displayed in Fig. 3.6. The intensities were corrected only for the dilution effect. Note, 550 nm is an isosbestic point for the absorption spectral changes that occur upon binding MC540 to LDL. Reprinted with permission from The Cancer Journal 1990; 3:360-365.

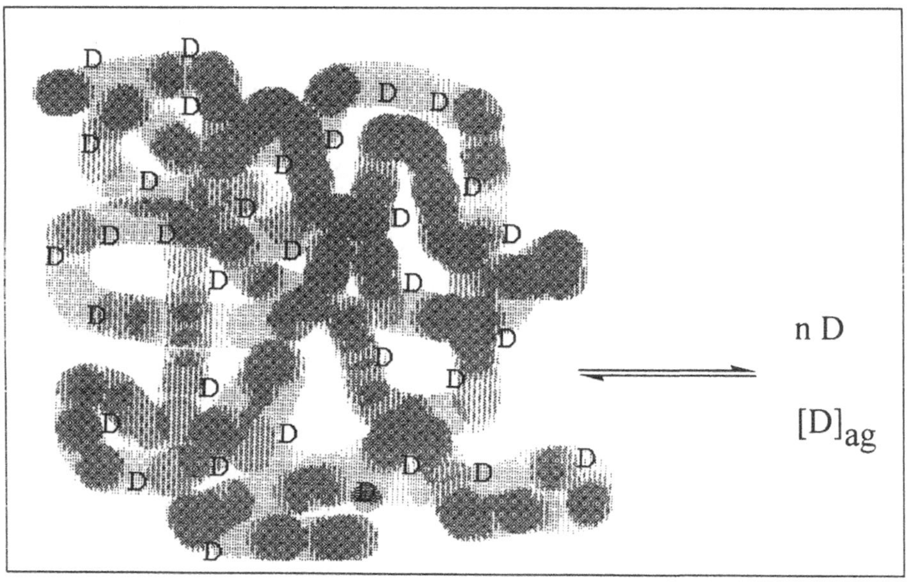

Fig. 3.8. Representation of the monomerization and uptake of dye (D) onto the surface of LDL. It should be stressed that the bound dye is highly fluorescent, in marked contrast to dye located in the aqueous phase where extensive aggegation takes place. It should also be noted that only dye bound to the protein can penetrate into intact biological cells. In the absence of protein, the dye adsorbs onto the external walls of the cell.

This secondary uptake occurs by way of displacement of lipid already bound to the protein. Binding of dye to lipoproteins provides the most effective means by which to incorporate the dye inside an intact biological cell.[7,8] In fact, in the absence of a carrier, MC540 does not assimilate into cells but simply deposits on the external cell walls.

The maximum concentration of MC540 that can be satisfactorily dissolved in water at pH 7 (with 50 mM sodium phosphate buffer) at 27°C containing 0.15 M NaCl is about 10 μM. At higher concentrations, there are undissolved aggregates of dye floating in the solution. Addition of LDL or ethanol causes complete dissolution of the aggregates and appearance of an absorption spectrum that is characteristic of the monomeric form of the dye.[6] Dissolution of the aggregate, with concomitant formation of the monomer, is most conveniently followed by fluorescence spectroscopy since, whereas the monomer is highly fluorescent, the aggregate is almost non-fluorescent (Fig. 3.8). This effect is well illustrated by the simple task of adding a small quantity of ethanol to an aqueous solution of MC540. The minimum amount of alcohol needed for complete monomerization of the dye is on the order of 25% by volume. The observed spectral changes are similar to those displayed in Figure 3.5.

A frequently used parameter in drug-related research is the partition coefficient, P. This term is usually taken as an indicator of the relative lipophilicity of the reagent and is measured by partitioning the drug against equal volumes of water and octanol; these two liquids being immiscible under ambient conditions. It is extremely important to have an understanding of the partition coefficient, because this often provides a simple measure of the solubility of the reagent within the targeted biological host. However, the conventional approach is not suitable for use with MC540 derivatives due to their poor solubility in water. Instead, we have devised an alternative method[3] in which the reagent is partitioned against chloroform and an aqueous solution of human serum albumin (Fig. 3.9). Under these conditions, MC540 partitions mostly to the aqueous phase, exhibiting a log P value of 1.18. This is a useful measure by which to compare the relative hydrophobicity of new derivatives and will be utilized extensively in later discussions.

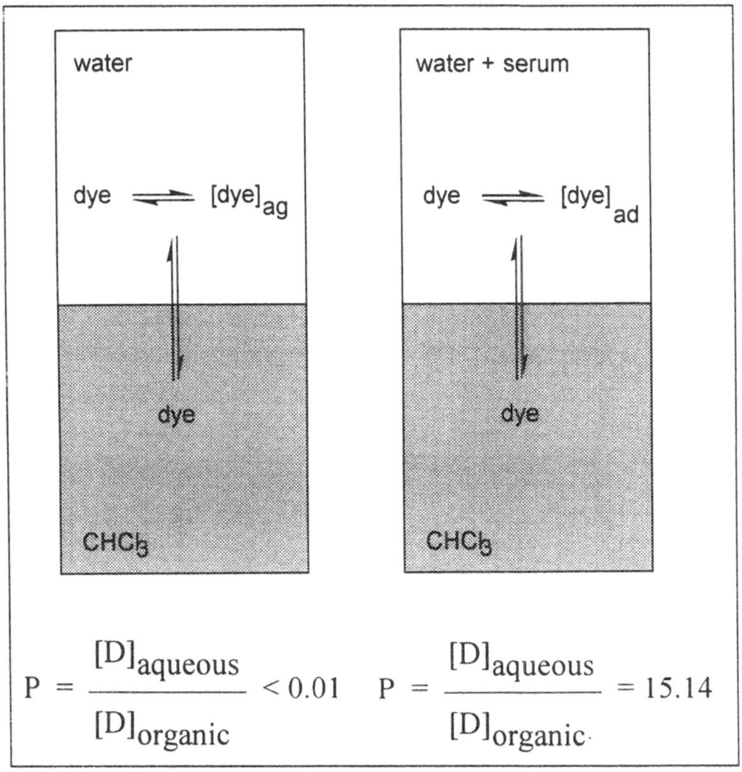

Fig. 3.9. Representation of the method used to measure partition coefficients for MC540 and its derivatives. Rather than use water to extract dye from an organic solvent, the method uses an aqueous solution of human serum albumin (2% w/w) since the dye has a very much higher affinity for protein than for water. The resultant concentrations of dye dissolved in each phase can be measured by absorption of fluorescence spectroscopy and compared to calibration charts.

Apart from its use in photography,[1] MC540 has been used extensively as a fluorescent probe for measuring membrane potentials.[9] This is made possible by the realization that the photophysical properties, especially the fluorescence quantum yield, are highly sensitive to the nature of the surrounding medium.[3,10-17] This effect was first described by Dixit and Mackay,[10] although the ability of MC540 to measure membrane potentials was already well known. The fluorescence lifetimes reported by Dixit and Mackay differ markedly from those recorded by later authors and, therefore, they have been omitted from Table 3.2. Also, the dependence of the fluorescence properties of MC540 on the local environment

Table 3.2 Effect of local environment on the fluorescence quantum yield (Φ_f) and excited singlet state lifetime (τ_s) of MC540, as measured at room temperature (See refs. 10-18 for more details.)

Medium	Φ_f	τ_s/ps
water	0.042	85
methanol	0.130	230
ethanol	0.160	410
pentanol	0.190	na
L1210[a]	0.140	650
HSA[b]	0.270	800
Triton X100[c]	0.310	840
SDS[d]	0.328	na
CTAB[e]	0.517	na
microemulsion[f]	0.504	na
glycerol	0.960	1450

(a) assimilated into L1210 leukemic cells, (b) bound to human serum albumin, (c) incorporated into Triton X100 neutral micelles dispersed in water, (d) sodium dodecylsulfonate micelles dispersed in water, (e) cetylammonium bromide micelles dispersed in water, (f) CTAB microemulsion.

was attributed to a micropolarity effect rather than being due to changes in viscosity, but later studies[3,15-17] showed that both polarity and viscosity influence the photophysical properties of merocyanine dyes.

Dixit and Mackay[10] further reported that illumination of MC540 in water with visible light resulted in rapid bleaching of the chromophore. Under identical conditions ($\lambda > 450$ nm), negligible bleaching (i.e. < 3%) occurred in alcohol solvents and micellar dispersions while no bleaching was observed in the microemulsion media. Removing the UV filter caused an increase in the rate of photobleaching but, even under such extreme conditions, there was no detectable degradation of the dye in microemulsion. Other researchers[15] have shown that MC540 bleaches in water, although the dye is extensively aggregated in the presence or absence of oxygen. Thus, photodegradation of the dye occurs by mechanisms other than those involving singlet molecular oxygen. It is important to note however, that degradation of MC540 can also be sensitized by singlet oxygen generating sensitizers.

When incorporated into lipid membranes, MC540 tends to associate near to the aqueous surface because of the sulfonic acid residue. In fact, if this group is fully dissociated the amount of energy required to bring it from the aqueous phase and immerse it in a nonpolar lipid membrane[9] would be on the order of 2,000 kJ mol^{-1}. In the absence of ion-pairing, therefore, the dye will not penetrate deep inside the membrane but will lie just below the surface. From computer molecular modeling studies, the length of the extended side-chain bearing the sulfonic acid residue is only ca. 0.60 nm. This localization of the dye near to the aqueous interface facilitates aggregation; the process being further assisted by the planar nature of the benzoxazole subunits (Fig. 3.10). Aggregation of this type results in extensive fluorescence quenching since the dye aggregate (or dimer!) is non-fluorescent. Ion-pairing with organic cations allows the dye to penetrate deeper into the membrane, although it is likely that most of the dye will remain close to the interface. It is also important to note that other types of dye aggregate can be formed, some of which are photoactive.[15]

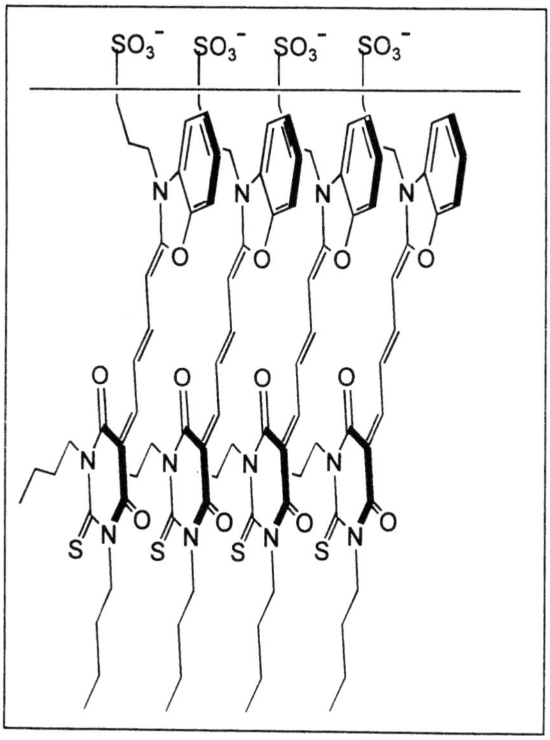

Fig. 3.10. Representation of the aggregate formed upon incorporation of MC540 into lipid membranes.

PHOTOPHYSICAL PROPERTIES OF MEROCYANINE 540

In alcohol solution, where the dye exists primarily as a monomeric species even at very high concentration, MC540 exhibits a sharp absorption band centered around 560 nm with a molar extinction coefficient in the region of 180,000 M^{-1} cm^{-1}. Excitation into this absorption band results in the appearance of fluorescence.[3] The fluorescence spectrum shows only a small Stokes shift, consistent with the excited singlet state retaining a similar (i.e. all *trans*) geometry to the ground state, with there being only a small change in polarity and good mirror symmetry with the absorption band (Fig. 3.11). By integration of the absorption band, the radioactive lifetime was calculated to be 2.7 ns, this being a typical value for a π,π^* excited singlet state. In ethanol solution at ambient temperature, the fluorescence quantum yield was measured to be 0.16 while the fluorescence lifetime, measured by time-resolved fluorescence spectroscopy with single-photon counting detection, was found to be 410 ps. Thus, the singlet lifetime is rather short,[3] indicating that the excited singlet state is unlikely to enter into bimolecular reactions unless the quencher is present in high concentration or positioned very close to the excited state.

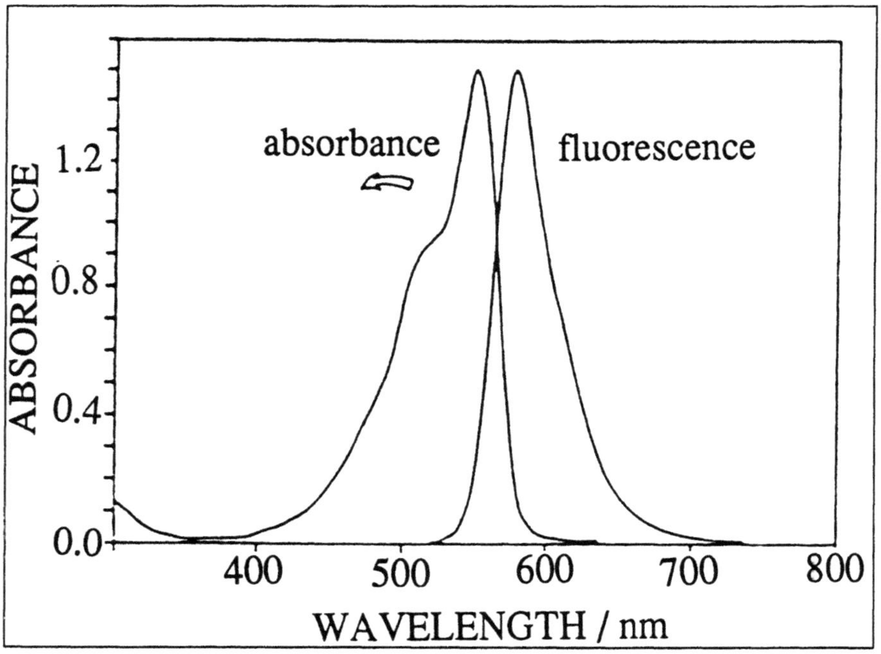

Fig. 3.11. Absorption and fluorescence spectra recorded for MC540 in ethanol solution at room temperature. Reprinted with permission from J Chem Soc Faraday Trans 1994; 90:953-961.

In fact, the diffusion-controlled bimolecular rate constant appropriate for ethanol solution at 20°C is 8.1 x 10^9 M^{-1} s^{-1} such that in order to effect 50% quenching of the excited singlet state it is necessary to employ a quencher concentration of ca. 0.3 M. A different way of expressing the same situation is to consider quenching of the excited singlet state by a small molecule having a (typical) diffusion coefficient of 5 x 10^{-6} cm^2 s^{-1}. In this case, the quencher can migrate about 0.65 nm within the period of the excited singlet state lifetime (Fig. 3.12). Quencher molecules lying outside this "critical distance" (which is not much larger than molecular contact!) will not be able to react with the excited state before it decays. In fact, rotation of large molecules like MC540 in ethanol at room temperature requires ca. 300 ps. Considering these factors in terms of a biological environment leads to the conclusion that only those dye molecules bound closely to a substrate will effect a chemical reaction under illumination. Consequently,

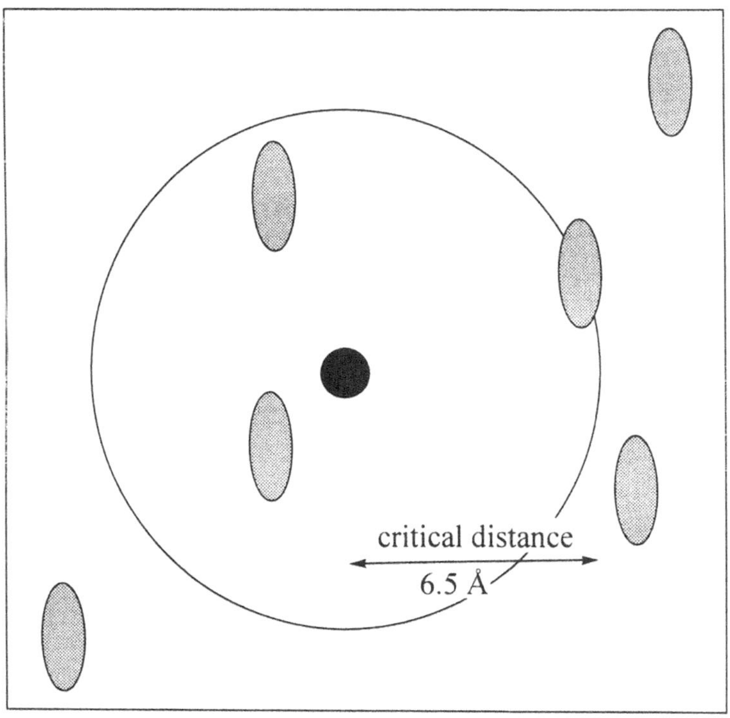

Fig. 3.12. Activated sphere model for fluorescence quenching. It is assumed that any quencher molecule lying within the critical distance of 6.5 Å will react with the excited state while quencher molecules residing outside this critical distance at the moment of excitation will not be able to react with the excited state.

binding of MC540 to a protein, enzyme or polynucleotide is essential if the excited singlet state is to function as the primary photosensitizer. While there is ample evidence to indicate that the dye binds avidly to proteins, MC540 shows little affinity for DNA, due in part to the presence of the water-solubilizing sulfonic acid residue.

The excited singlet state can also be monitored by transient absorption spectroscopy following excitation of the dye with a 30 ps laser pulse at 532 nm. Under such conditions,[16] the incident laser pulse causes transient bleaching of the intense ground state absorption band centered at 560 nm and the concomitant appearance of a rather weak absorption signal located slightly to the blue of the ground state absorption band (Fig. 3.13). This transient absorption signal arises from absorption by the excited singlet state and, by time resolving the process, it is evident that the signal decays at exactly the same rate as monitored by fluorescence spectroscopy. Also apparent in the transient absorption spectrum is the occurrence of stimulated emission. This latter process appears as an intense fluorescence spectrum as induced by absorption of photons from the monitoring laser pulse. Again, the signal due to stimulated emission decays at the same rate as found for normal fluorescence, indicating that a single species is responsible for all three processes.

Examination of the laser flash photolysis records on slower time scales[3,15,17] shows the presence of an additional two transients that persist after decay of the excited singlet state. In fact, it is clear that these two transient species are formed exclusively from the excited singlet state. The transients exhibit quite disparate differential absorption spectra and survive for different periods (Fig. 3.14). The shorter-lived species reacts rapidly with molecular oxygen introduced into the solution and, therefore, can be assigned to the triplet excited state of the dye. In deoxygenated ethanol solution, the triplet state has a lifetime of ca. 820 μs—a factor of 2 million-fold with respect to the corresponding excited singlet state. The second transient, which has a lifetime of 6.7 ms in ethanol at room temperature, does not react with molecular oxygen and is attributed to an unstable geometric isomer formed via rotation around one of the double bonds in the polymethine bridge. The rates of formation and decay of this isomer are markedly dependent on the viscosity of the surrounding medium, as might be

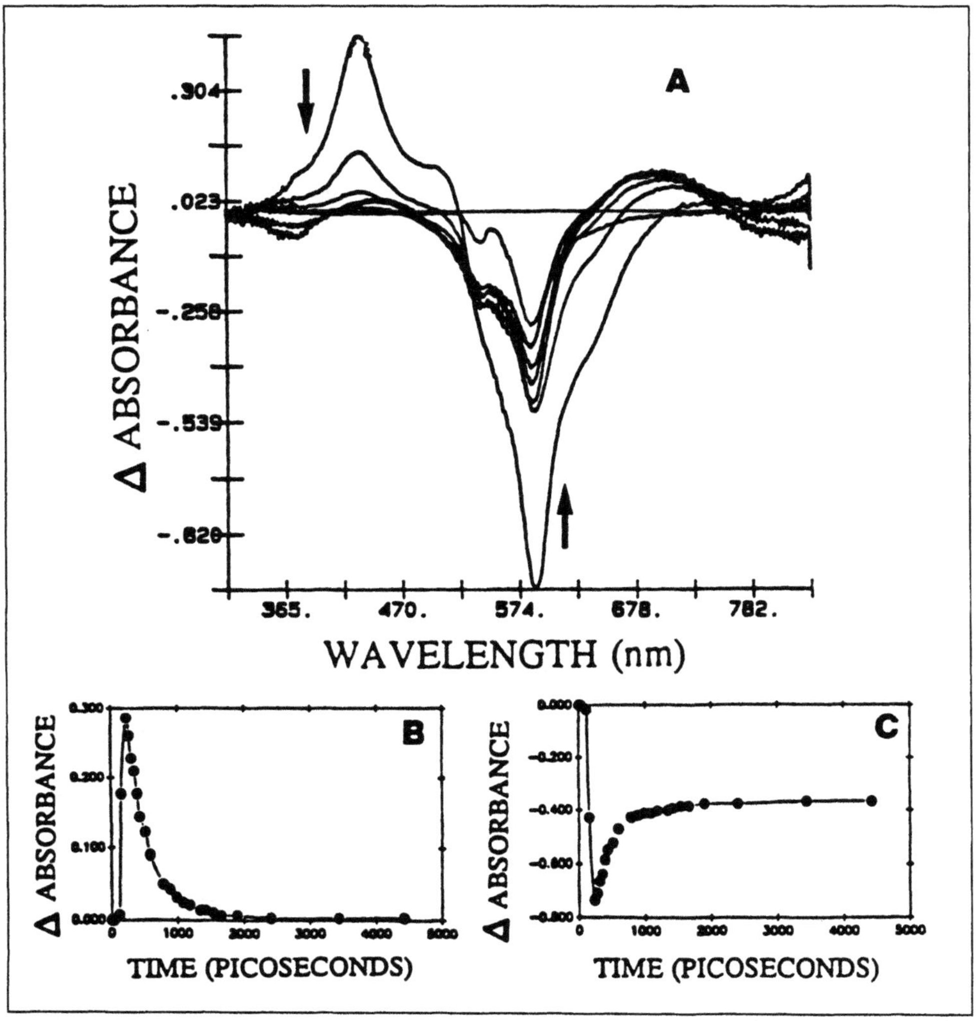

*Fig. 3.13. (A) Transient absorption spectra recorded after excitation of merocyanine **2** in methanol solution with a 30 ps laser pulse at 532 nm: delay times were 0, 0.45, 1.0, 2.0, 3.5, 5.0 and 6.0 ns after the laser pulse. Decay profiles were measured at (B) 440 nm where the excited singlet state shows pronounced absorption and (C) 590 nm where the ground state absorbs. Note the incomplete recovery of the ground state shown in (C) that occurs on this time scale due to formation of the excited triplet state and the cis-isomer.Reprinted with permission from J Photochem Photobiol, A Chem 1992; 65:79-93.*

expected for a process involving large-scale torsional motion.[3] By considering all the available spectroscopic evidence, together with molecular modeling studies, it is concluded that the isomer is the *cis* form generated by way of rotation of the benzoxazole subunit about the central double bond (see Structure 3.6).

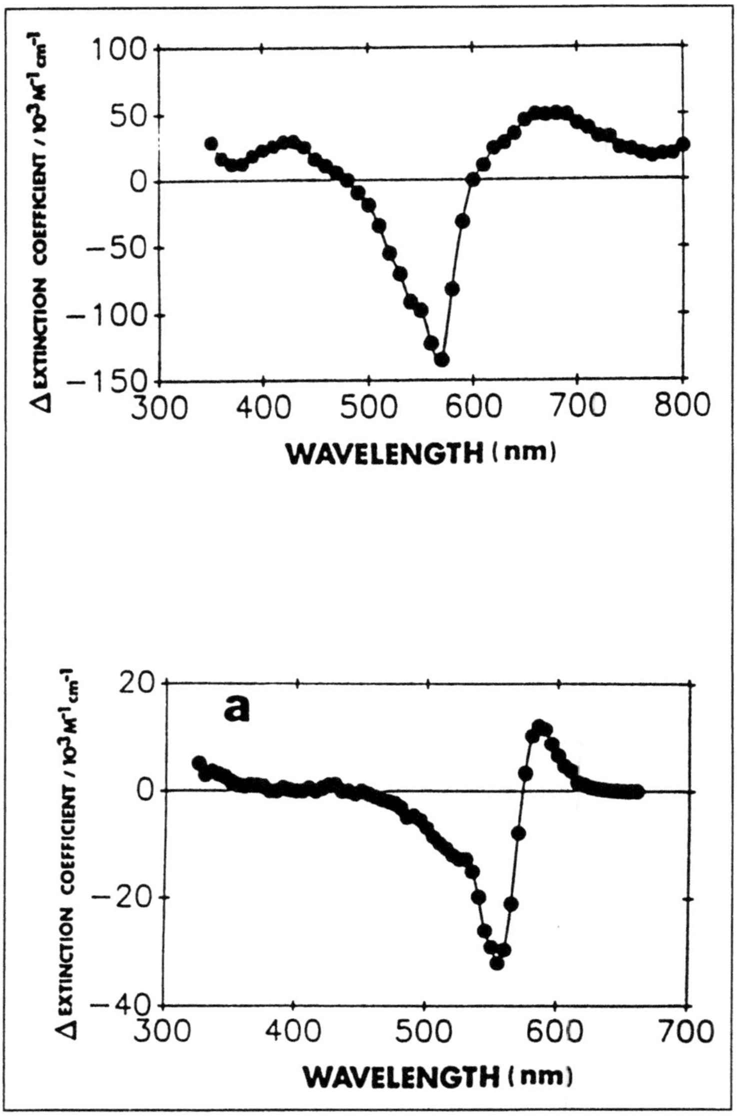

Fig. 3.14. (a) Differential absorption spectrum recorded for the triplet excited state of MC540 in deoxygenated methanol as generated by triplet energy transfer from anthracene. (b) Differential absorption spectrum recorded for the unstable cis-isomer of MC540 as formed by laser flash photolysis in oxygen-saturated methanol. Reprinted with permission from Photochem Photobiol 1991; 53:1-11.

The *cis* isomer reverts back to the original *trans* isomer[3,17] in a thermal process (Structure 3.7) for which there is a large activation energy and for which the overall enthalpy change is 75 kJ mol^{-1}. Indeed, by measuring the rate of (dark) conversion of the *cis* isomer to the *trans* isomer in ethanol as a function of temperature the activation energy was found to be 120 kJ mol^{-1}. The corresponding barrier for thermal isomerization of the *trans* isomer is far too high for this process to take place in ethanol solution, even under reflux, and only a single geometric form persists in solution

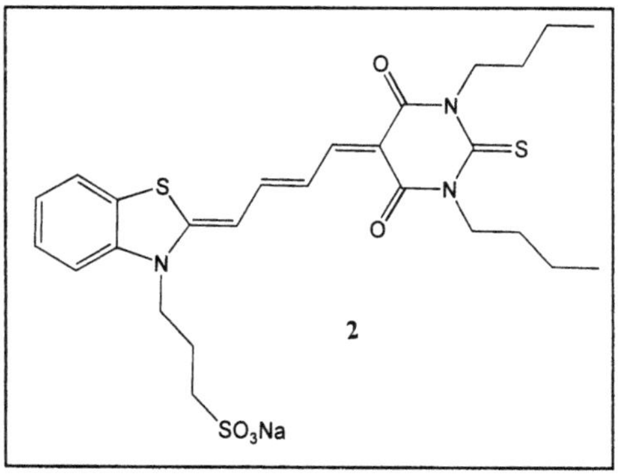

*Structure 3.6. Structure of the thio-derivative **2** of MC540.*

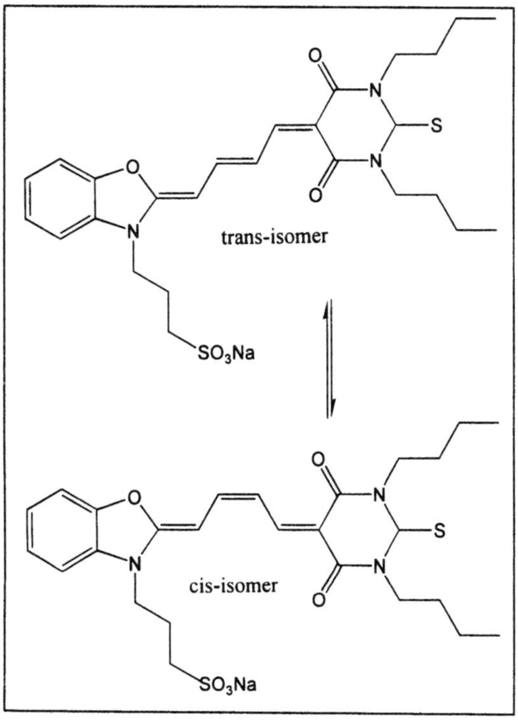

Structure 3.7. Interconversion of trans and cis isomers.

at room temperature in the dark. The *cis* isomer has an absorption spectrum remarkably similar to that of the corresponding *trans* isomer (Fig. 3.15) and, consequently, absorbs incident photons intended to excite the *trans* form. In fact, the *cis* isomer is extremely photoactive and decays rapidly under illumination. In part, this photoreaction results in bleaching of the chromophore, even in the complete absence of molecular oxygen.

In marked contrast to the thermal (dark) isomerization process, light-induced formation of the *cis* isomer involves a much

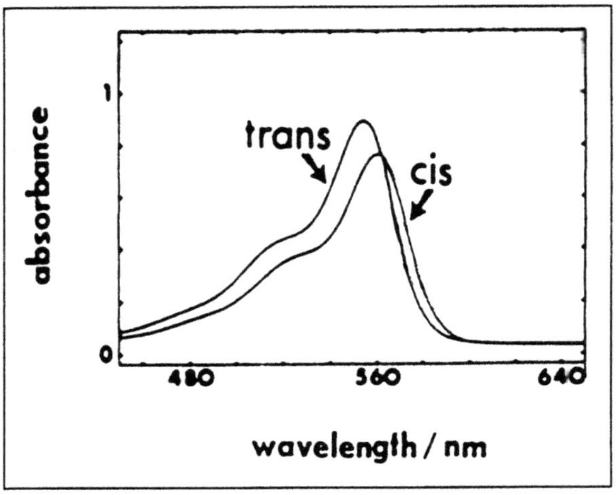

Fig. 3.15. Comparison of absorption spectra recorded for the trans- and cis-isomers of MC540 in ethanol solution. Reprinted with permission from Photochem Photobiol 1991; 53:1-11.

smaller activation energy. By measuring the rate of formation of this species in ethanol as a function of temperature it was concluded[3,17] that the activation barrier for photoisomerization of the *trans* isomer to the corresponding *cis* isomer is only 24 kJ mol^{-1}. Photoisomerization is, in fact, the major deactivation route for the excited singlet state of MC540 in ethanol solution at 20°C and accounts for about 40% of the photon balance under such conditions. These various realizations allow construction of a potential energy level diagram (Fig. 3.16) that accounts for the photophysical properties of MC540 in alcohol solvents. Thus, excitation of the ground state *trans* isomer populates the π,π^* excited singlet state that retains a very similar geometric structure. The singlet excited state may fluoresce or undergo intersystem crossing to generate the corresponding π,π^* excited triplet state, which also possesses the all *trans* geometry. In competition to radioactive decay and intersystem crossing, the singlet excited state can undergo isomerization by way of a planar transition state (TS). This transition state, which will be in an excited singlet state configuration, undergoes rapid internal conversion to form the highly unstable ground state transition state. This latter species undergoes nuclear displacement to form a mixture of *trans* and *cis* isomers with the *cis* isomer slowly reverting to the *trans* isomer in the dark. Before considering the factors that combine to control the rates of these isomerization processes it is worthwhile reflecting on the competitive formation of the π,π^* excited triplet state.

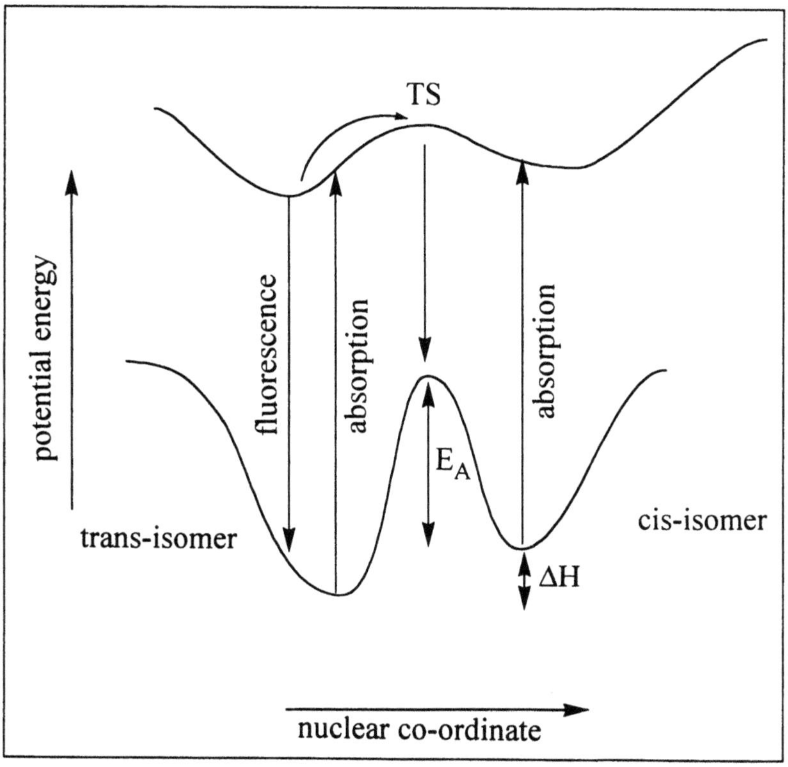

Fig. 3.16. Potential energy diagram illustrating the photoisomerization of MC540 in ethanol solution.

In deoxygenated ethanol at 20°C the excited triplet state of MC540 is formed in extremely low quantum yield; detailed investigations[3] place this value at ca. 0.003. The triplet does not phosphoresce, even in an ethanol glass at 77 K, but is readily detected by its characteristic differential absorption spectrum. Although present in low yield, the triplet state possesses a relatively long lifetime and, consequently, a much larger active sphere for reaction than that shown by the much shorter-lived excited singlet state (Figs. 3.17 and 3.18). Indeed, the triplet state is quenched at the diffusion controlled bimolecular rate limit by molecular oxygen resulting in formation of singlet molecular oxygen, $O_2(^1\Delta_g)$. Of course, the quantum yield for generation of $O_2(^1\Delta_g)$ must necessarily be very low since it cannot exceed the quantum yield for formation of the triplet state itself. Furthermore, $O_2(^1\Delta_g)$, which possesses a lifetime of ca. 12 μs in ethanol solution, reacts irreversibly with ground state MC540 to produce a variety of breakdown

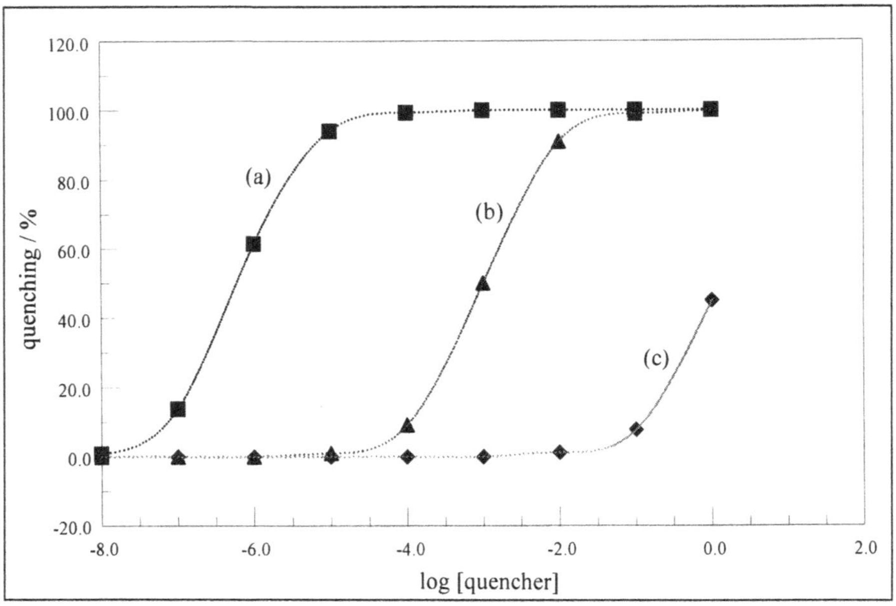

Fig. 3.17. (a) Correlation between the extent of triplet state quenching by molecular oxygen (expressed as a percentage) and the concentration of oxygen, assuming quenching takes place with a bimolecular rate constant of 2 x 10^9 M^{-1} s^{-1} in ethanol at room temperature. For comparative purposes the quenching efficiency is also shown for oxygen reacting with (b) the triplet state in a lipid bilayer membrane and (c) the singlet excited state in ethanol.

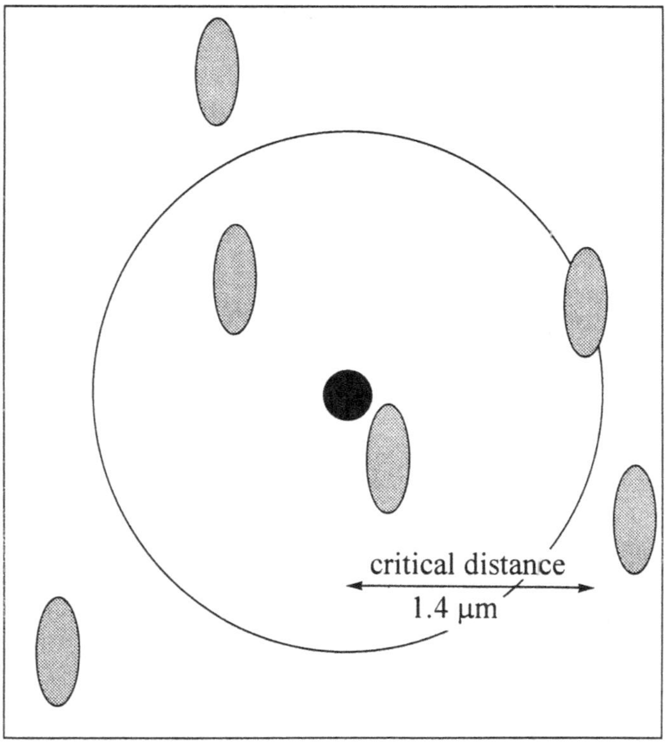

Fig. 3.18. Activated sphere model for triplet state quenching by molecular oxygen. It is assumed that an oxygen molecule lying within the critical distance of 1.4 μm will react with the excited triplet state while oxygen molecules residing outside this critical distance at the moment of excitation will not be able to react with the triplet.

products. The overall bimolecular rate constant for interaction between $O_2(^1\Delta_g)$ and MC540, which clearly includes contributions from physical (i.e. vibrational) quenching and chemical reaction, is $2.1 \times 10^9\ M^{-1}\ s^{-1}$ in ethanol at ambient temperature (Scheme 3.1). The formal quantum yield for bleaching of ground state MC540 by $O_2(^1\Delta_g)$ under these conditions was measured to be ca. 0.0001.

Evidently, there is a major stumbling block to the development of effective PDT-type photosensitizers based on MC540. While the singlet excited state, formed with unitary quantum yield, is too short-lived to react with constituents of the biomaterial other than by direct binding, the triplet state, being long-lived and readily available for slow diffusional bimolecular reactions, is populated in too low quantum yield for it to be a viable photosensitizer. The problem relates to the very efficient photoisomerization that occurs from the excited singlet state of the dye. Light-induced isomerization in itself might be a useful property since it provides access to unique structural features that might figure in the all-important recognition mechanism—without selective recognition of and assimilation into infected cells there is no purpose whatsoever in proposing a compound as a therapeutic reagent. It is possible that the *cis* isomer assists in the recognition process (see later) while it must be recalled that the *cis* isomer is itself highly photoactive. Thus, in situ generation of the *cis* isomer might be the means by which MC540 produces an efficacious photosensitizer. It is necessary to bear in mind at all times that photoisomerization to the *cis* isomer is always the single most important process that occurs for MC540 under illumination.

In order to further explore the mechanics of the isomerization processes, the rate of isomerization was monitored as a function of viscosity and polarity of the surrounding medium.[3,16,17] Both light-induced (*trans* to *cis*) and dark (*cis* to *trans*) isomerization steps were found to be affected by the viscosity of the solvent and by the polarity of the medium. These effects were studied in considerable detail for the corresponding merocyanine dye formed from benzthiazole, 2. The overall activation energy associated with isomerization (E_A) can be partitioned into individual terms relating to the viscosity (E_V) and polarity (E_P) of the surrounding medium, as well as a term associated with rotation around the central double bond (E_R):

$$E_A = E_V + E_R - E_P \tag{2}$$

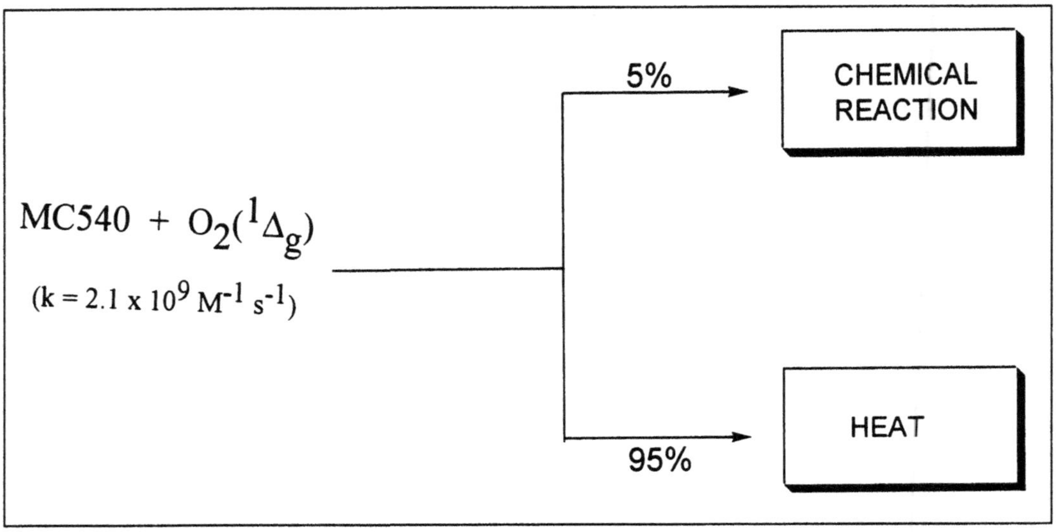

Scheme 3.1. Partitioning of the interaction between the triplet excited state of MC540 and molecular oxygen in ethanol solution.

In summary, the viscosity dependence, which is more correctly formulated in terms of microviscosity, arises because isomerization involves frictional forces between dye and surrounding solvent molecules. Solvent molecules must be displaced in order for isomerization to proceed and microviscosity provides a crude estimate of frictional forces between solvent molecules in the reservoir. The polarity effect is caused because of the zwitterionic nature of MC540 which provides for a dipole moment across the molecule (Structure 3.8). This zwitterionic character affects the bond order of carbon atoms in the polyene bridge such that the formal alternating bond orders of one and two approach the limiting value of 1.5 as the solvent polarity increases. A lower bond order promotes isomerization by way of reducing the activation energy. The polarity-dependent activation energy is conveniently expressed in terms of the solvent $E_T(30)$ parameter

$$E_V = \beta\ [E_T(30) - 30] \times 4.18 \qquad (3)$$

where the b parameter has values of 0.11 and -0.09, respectively, for the photoinduced and thermal isomerization processes.

Because of this interplay between viscosity and polarity, it is extremely difficult to predict the photophysical properties of MC540 in a different medium. Thus, attempts to predict the photophysical properties of the dye after assimilation into an in-

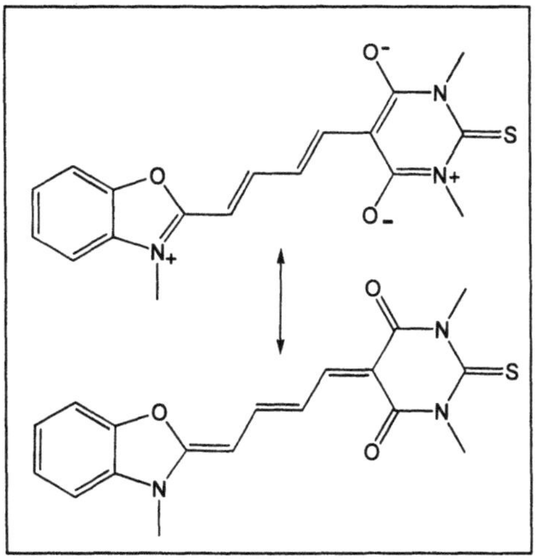

Structure 3.8. Polar and nonpolar forms of MC540.

tact biological cell are hazardous and it must be stressed that the extreme sensitivity of these properties to the nature of the environment mean that, in all probability, a wide variety of photophysical properties will be available for in situ localized MC540. Each different location will be characterized by unique photophysical properties.

Finally, it is interesting to consider what would be the optimal conditions for maximizing the triplet quantum yield and to inquire as to what this optimal value might be! In the event that restricting photoisomerization would result in an enhanced triplet quantum yield we can easily identify the environmental factors that control isomerization. Thus, increasing the viscosity of the surrounding medium would inhibit photoisomerization. From the measured "viscosity-related activation energy" of 9.2 kJ mol^{-1}, we can estimate that the triplet quantum yield in ethanol at a viscosity of 30 cP, as might be expected in a lipid membrane, would be ca. 0.008. Similarly, the transition state is more polar than is the excited singlet state such that polar solvents increase the rate of photoisomerization (but decrease the rate of thermal isomerization). The "polarity-related activation energy" is quite high, such that decreasing the solvent polarity should serve to increase the triplet quantum yield. Again, extrapolating the polarity to that expected for a lipid membrane (i.e. $E_T \approx 30$) results in an estimate for the triplet quantum yield of ca. 0.015. Completely restricting photoisomerization would result in a triplet quantum yield of only

0.02. This is hardly conducive with the notion of MC540 being an effective triplet state photosensitizer, even if appropriate conditions for its realization could be achieved. Instead, in order to improve these photosensitizing properties it seems necessary to synthesize alternative derivatives that might exhibit more attractive photophysical properties.

ENHANCING THE TRIPLET QUANTUM YIELD

The inherent quantum yield for formation of the triplet excited state of MC540 in fluid media is far too low for the compound to be proposed as a triplet state photosensitizer, unless the reagent possesses some remarkably significant selective recognition properties. Apart from controlling the nature of the environment, there are two easy ways to influence the yield of the triplet state and thereby convert a poor photosensitizer into a much more effective one. First, the rate of photoisomerization can be reduced by increasing the size of the isomerizing subunits since the rate is expected to decrease with increasing volume of the rotor (Structure 3.9). Second, the rate of intersystem crossing from excited singlet state to the triplet manifold might be increased by incorporation into the structure of atoms having large spin-orbital coupling constants. The latter atoms might be halogens or heteroatoms of high atomic number.

Our first approach[3] towards varying the size of the rotating groups concerned the synthesis of MC540 derivatives having different alkyl groups attached to the amido N atoms of the barbiturate subunit. These compounds display the same basic type

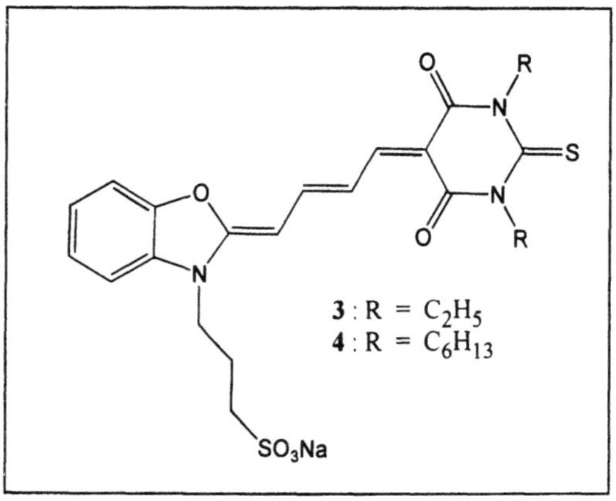

Structure 3.9. A simple means for changing the molar volume of MC540.

(i.e. fluorescence, triplet formation and isomerization) of photophysical behavior as outlined for MC540 in deoxygenated ethanol solution (Figs. 3.19 and 3.20). The derived photophysical properties are collected in Table 3.3. In particular, the absorption and fluorescence spectra remain comparable to those of MC540 (Fig. 3.19) with the absorption maximum (λ_{max}) being fixed

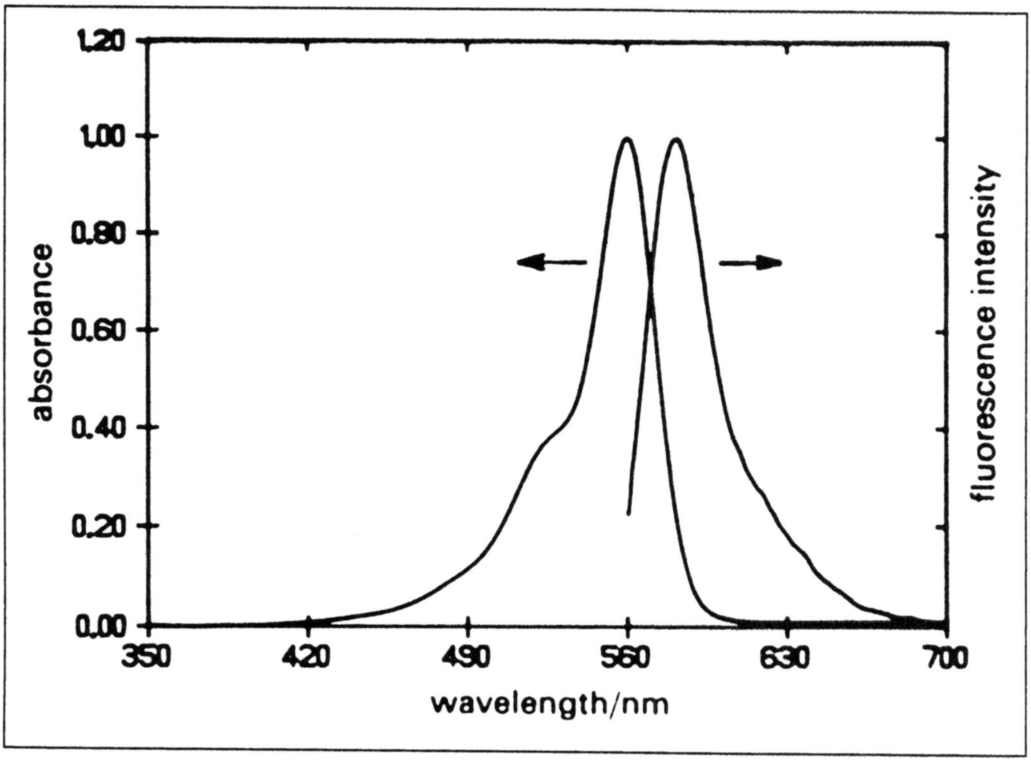

*Fig. 3.19. Absorption and fluorescence spectra recorded for merocyanine **1** in dilute ethanol solution. The excitation wavelength used for the fluorescence spectrum was 540 nm. Reprinted with permission from J Chem Soc Faraday Trans 1994; 90:953-961.*

Table 3.3. Photophysical properties measured for merocyanine dyes of differing molar volume in dilute ethanol solution (See ref. 3 for more details.)

Compound	λ_{max}/nm	Φ_f	τ_s/ps	Φ_t	$\tau_t/\mu s$	Φ_i	τ_i/ms
1	560	0.170	380	0.0030	210	0.47	3.7
3	560	0.163	430	0.0035	775	0.42	6.9
MC540	560	0.160	410	0.0030	820	0.40	6.7
4	560	0.170	415	0.0031	495	0.45	6.1
5	572	0.092	530	0.0038	780	0.24	42.0
6	601	0.024	380	0.0072	750	0.12	52.0

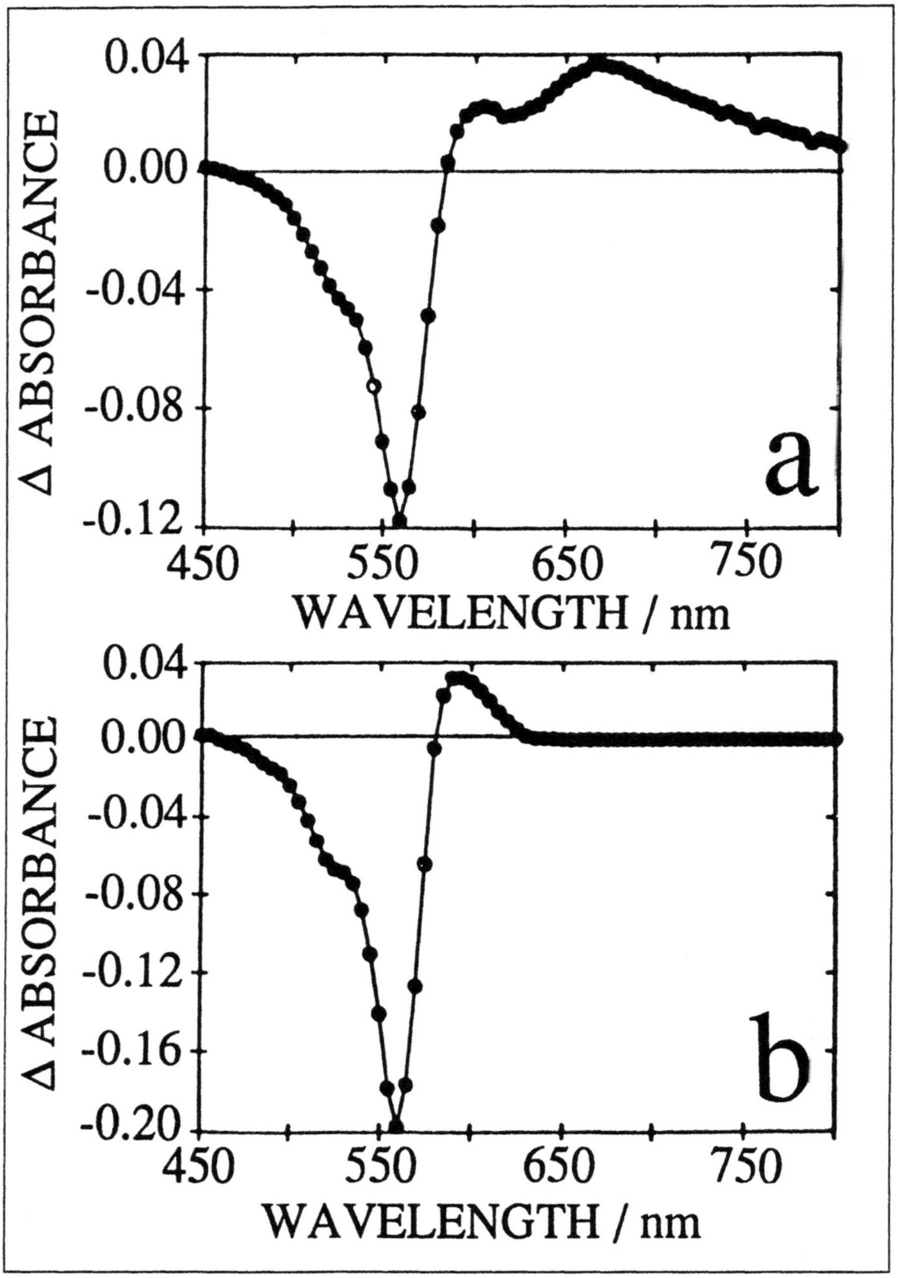

*Fig. 3.20. Differential absorption spectra recorded 1 µs after excitation of merocyanine **1** in (a) deoxygenated and (b) oxygen-saturated ethanol solution with a 10 ps laser pulse at 532 nm. Panel (a) contains contributions from both excited triplet state and the unstable cis-isomer while panel (b) shows the spectrum for the isomer alone. Reprinted with permission from J Chem Soc Faraday Trans 1994; 90:953-961.*

at ca. 560 nm. The fluorescence quantum yields (Φ_f) and excited singlet state lifetimes (τ_s) are not sensitive to the size of the alkyl groups, while the quantum yields for formation of the triplet excited state (Φ_t) and of the *cis* isomer (Φ_i) show little, if any, dependence on the molar volume of the rotor. Small variations in the triplet lifetime (τ_t) and in the lifetime of the unstable *cis* isomer (τ_i) confirm the insensitivity of the photophysical properties of this set of derivatives towards the size of the rotating group. Such behavior is consistent with the thiobarbiturate subunit remaining almost motionless during photoisomerization and also during the subsequent thermal step. This situation might be expected if hydrogen bonding between the carbonyl groups and hydrogen atoms in the polymethine chain effectively locked the thiobarbiturate unit into place. As such, changing the length of the alkyl substituents has little real effect on the overall photophysical properties of the dye.

If correct, this hypothesis can be used to infer that the benzoxazole subunit is the one that is displaced during isomerization. In this case, the molar volume of the rotor can be varied by changing the length of the chain bearing the water-solubilizing group or by fusing additional aromatic residues to the periphery of the benzoxazole subunit. It should be noted that replacing the sulfonate group with a methyl group, forming compound **1**, tends to decrease the molar volume and is accompanied by a slight increase in the rate of isomerization. More significantly, increasing the size of the benzoxazole subunit (Structure 3.10) causes a major decrease in the rate of isomerization that is accompanied by concomitant increases in fluorescence and triplet quantum yields. Unfortunately, the yield of the triplet state remains at a very low level and it is clear that this is not a useful strategy for improving the efficacy for triplet sensitization. It should also be noted that these various synthetic adaptations cause large changes in the physical properties of the dye, especially the solubility in water and the partition coefficient.

It is possible to decrease the yield of the unstable *cis* isomer by including bulky groups into the polyene bridge.[18] Thus, a small set of appropriately modified derivatives (Structure 3.11) was synthesized. Here, the quantum yields for formation of the *cis* isomer were measured in ethanol solution following laser excitation at 532 nm (Table 3.4). It is seen that building the polymethine bridge into a cyclohexenyl ring has the effect of completely inhibiting

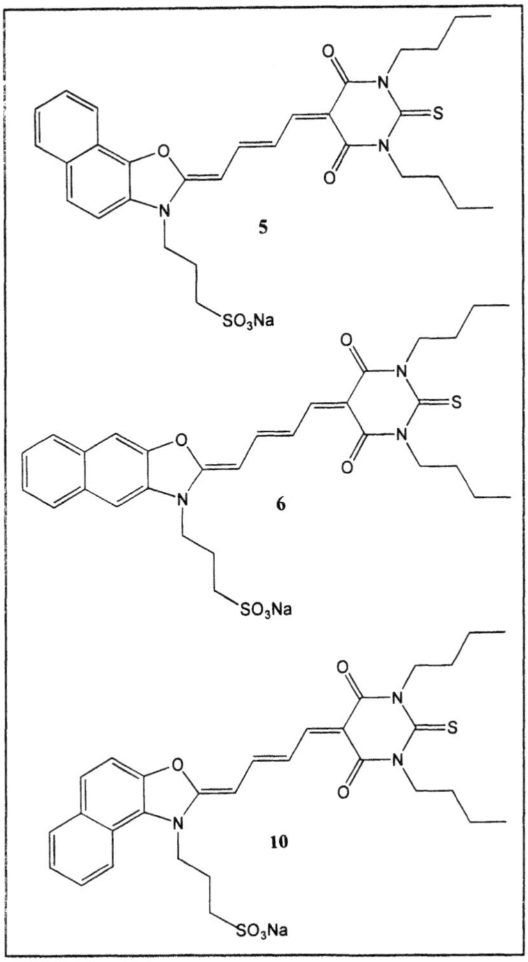

Structure 3.10. Increasing the size and stereochemistry of the head group.

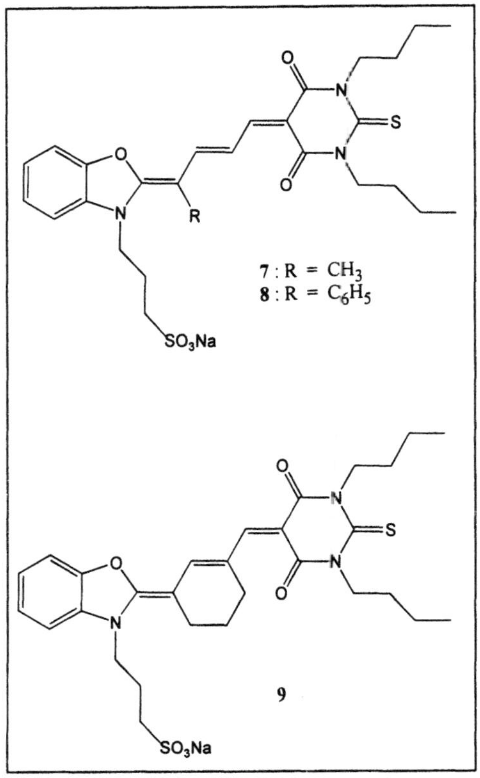

Structure 3.11. Incorporating blocking groups into the polyene chain.

Table 3.4. Photophysical properties measured for merocyanine dyes having bulky groups inserted into the polymethine bridge

Compound	λ_{max}/nm	Φ_f	τ_s/ps	Φ_t	τ_t/µs	Φ_i	τ_i / ms
MC540	560	0.160	410	0.0030	820	0.40	6.7
7	561	0.022	280	0.0010	880	0.17	22.5
8	565	0.028	290	0.0016	560	0.12	18.7
9	567	0.037	185	0.0002	850	<0.01	nd

nd—not detected

isomerization. However, this effect is not accompanied by a reasonable increase in triplet yield. Clearly, such substituents tend to increase the rate of internal conversion, because of distortions to the ground state structure, notably the degree of planarity, without affecting the rate of isomerization.

More significant changes in the photophysical properties become available by incorporating different heteroatoms into the structural skeleton (Table 3.5). This can be done rather easily by replacing the oxygen atom in the benzoxazole subunit with carbon, sulfur or selenium and/or by replacing the terminal sulfur atom in the thiobarbiturate subunit with oxygen or selenium (Structure 3.12). The overall strategy gives rise to a large series of derivatives that differ only in respect of the nature of the

Table 3.5. Photophysical properties measured for merocyanine dyes of different heteroatoms incorporated into the molecular skeleton (Data for merocyanines* 6 *and* 14 *are taken from ref. 22. All other data are from ref. 21.)

Compound	λ_{max}/nm	Φ_f	τ_s/ps	Φ_t	τ_t/μs	Φ_i	τ_i / ms
MC540	560	0.160	410	0.003	820	0.40	6.7
5	572	0.180	530	0.0038	780	0.24	42.0
6	601	0.004	na	< 0.01	na	na	na
11	592	0.180	660	0.003	800	0.37	1.0
2	595	0.180	780	0.008	670	0.31	1.2
12	604	0.180	700	0.100	135	0.05	2.4
13	535	0.150	370	0.0017	180	0.51	3.1
14	561	0.012	na	0.80	18	0.19	na
15	602	0.008	70	0.55	95	0.02	3.5

na – not available

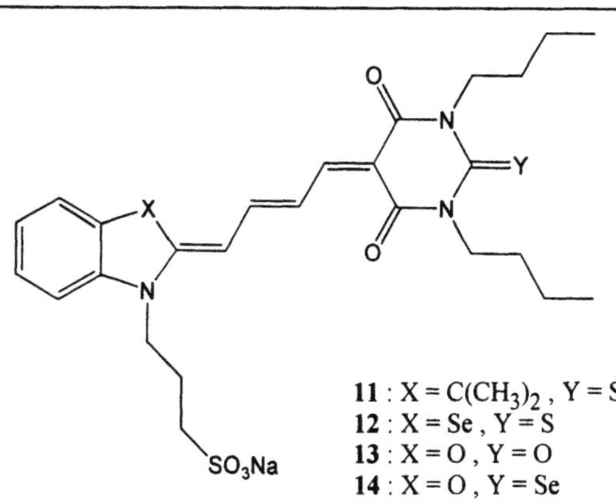

11 : X = $C(CH_3)_2$, Y = S
12 : X = Se , Y = S
13 : X = O , Y = O
14 : X = O , Y = Se
15 : X = Se , Y = Se

Structure 3.12. Varying the nature of the heteroatoms.

heteroatoms.[19-21] Examination of the photophysical data[21] shows that the quantum yield for formation of the triplet excited state can be varied over an extremely wide range using this synthetic approach. Of course, the "internal heavy-atom effect", which is the generic name for this kind of spin-orbital coupling perturbation, does not only operate on intersystem crossing from excited singlet state to triplet manifold but it also catalyses nonradiative deactivation of the excited triplet state. Thus, in addition to promoting formation of the triplet state, heavy-atoms like selenium will also shorten the triplet lifetime. The experimental results, however, indicate that this is not too severe a problem and the triplet lifetime remains reasonably long throughout this series of compounds. Indeed, in each case the triplet lifetime is sufficiently long for this excited state to react quantitatively with molecular oxygen in aerated ethanol solution.

In O_2-saturated ethanol at room temperature the various triplet excited states react with molecular oxygen to produce singlet molecular oxygen, $O_2(^1\Delta_g)$. The quantum yields for generation of $O_2(^1\Delta_g)$ closely follow the relative order of triplet quantum yields, again showing that this strategy allows the photochemical properties of the dye to be manipulated over a very wide range. It has further been shown by Günter et al[19,20] that the ability of merocyanine dyes to photoeradicate viruses and to inactivate leukemic cells depends markedly on the nature of the heteroatoms incorporated into the molecular backbone. The inference, clearly, is that there might be a correlation between biocidal activity and ability to generate $O_2(^1\Delta_g)$ in fluid solution.[22] We will return to this point a little later in the discussion.

ELECTRON TRANSFER REACTIONS

Davila et al first reported[17] clear evidence indicating that MC540 could participate in light-induced electron transfer reactions with adventitious redox partners. Thus, it was observed that the singlet excited state of MC540 was quenched by 2-methyl-1,4-benzoquinone (MBQ) in methanol solution at the diffusion-controlled rate limit ($k = 2.1 \times 10^{10}$ M^{-1} s^{-1}). Identical fluorescence quenching behavior was observed when reaction was followed by steady-state or dynamic fluorescence spectroscopy (Fig. 3.21) showing that the reaction does not require formation of a ground state complex. The triplet excited state is also quenched by MBQ

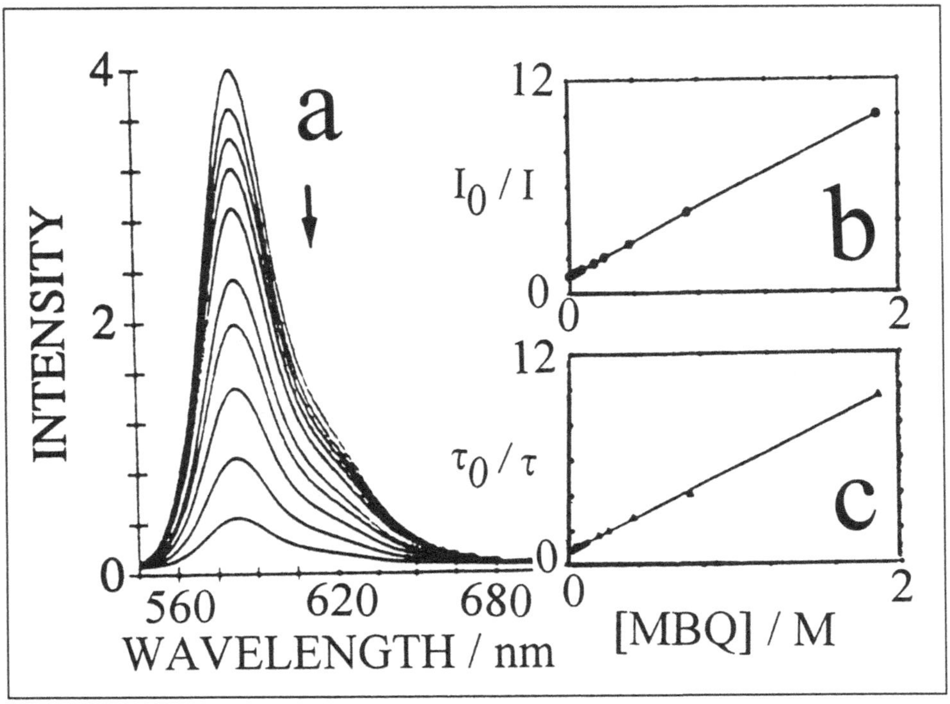

Fig. 3.21. (a) Decrease in fluorescence observed upon addition of increasing amounts of MBQ to MC540 in methanol. (b) The fluorescence quenching data presented in the form of a Stern-Vollmer plot; and (c) the corresponding Stern-Vollmer plot observed from fluorescence lifetime measurements. Reprinted with permission from Photochem Photobiol 1991; 53:1-11.

($k = 5.8 \times 10^9\ M^{-1}\ s^{-1}$) in the absence of oxygen. Laser flash photolysis studies indicated that these quenching reactions resulted in net electron transfer to form the corresponding π-radical ions (Fig. 3.22).

$$MC540^* + MBQ \rightarrow MC540^{+\cdot} + MBQ^{-\cdot} \quad (4)$$

The resultant p-radical cation of MC540 formed by electron transfer to the quinone reacts with hydroquinone ($MBQH_2$) present as an impurity.

$$MC540^{+\cdot} + MBQH_2 \rightarrow MC540 + MBQ^{-\cdot} + 2H^+ \quad (5)$$

$$2MBQ^{-\cdot} + 2H^+ \rightarrow MBQ + MBQH_2 \quad (6)$$

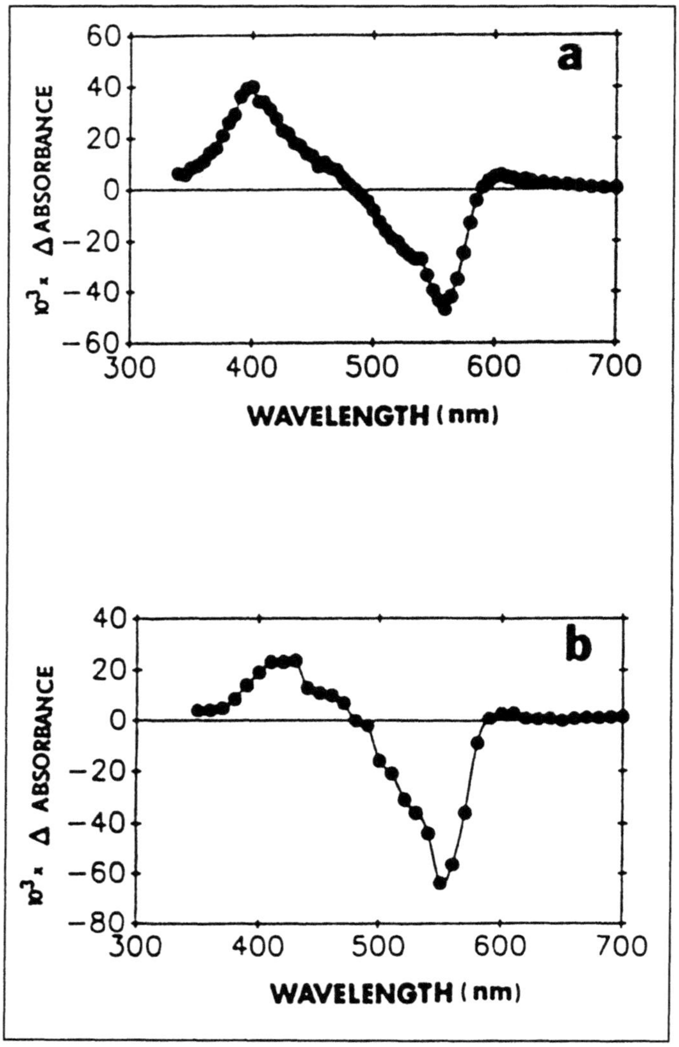

Fig. 3.22. Transient differential absorption spectra recorded 100 ns after laser excitation of MC540 in deoxygenated methanol containing 1 M (a) methyl viologen; and (b) 2-methyl-1,4-benzoquinone. Reprinted with permission from Photochem Photobiol 1991; 53:1-11.

The fluorescence of MC540 in methanol solution was also quenched by methyl viologen (MV^{2+}). Again, quenching occurred at the diffusion-controlled rate limit ($k = 3.1 \times 10^{10}\ M^{-1}\ s^{-1}$), allowing for electrostatic attraction between the reactants. The triplet excited state of MC540 was quenched by the viologen ($k = 2.6 \times 10^{10}\ M^{-1}\ s^{-1}$) at almost the same rate, indicating that the reaction is very much thermodynamically allowed. Laser flash photolysis studies[17] confirmed the intermediate formation of π-radical ions (Fig. 3.22).

$$MC540^{*} + MV^{2+} \rightarrow MC540^{+\cdot} + MV^{+\cdot} \qquad (7)$$

In this case, the π-radical ions recombined to restore the ground state system with a bimolecular rate constant of 7 x 10^9 M^{-1} s^{-1}. Unlike the electron transfer reaction observed with quinone, this system is fully reversible.

$$MC540^{+\cdot} + MV^{+\cdot} \rightarrow MC540 + MV^{2+} \quad (8)$$

It has also been reported that MC540 can be reduced under illumination in the presence of electron donors such as glutathione, cysteine or NADPH provided oxygen is removed from the solution.[23] The reduced form of MC540 is able to transfer an electron to certain nitroxide spin traps. Subsequent studies[3] using pulse radiolysis techniques confirmed that MC540 was readily reduced by appropriate one-electron reductants and allowed spectroscopic detection of the intermediate π-radical anion (Fig. 3.23). This

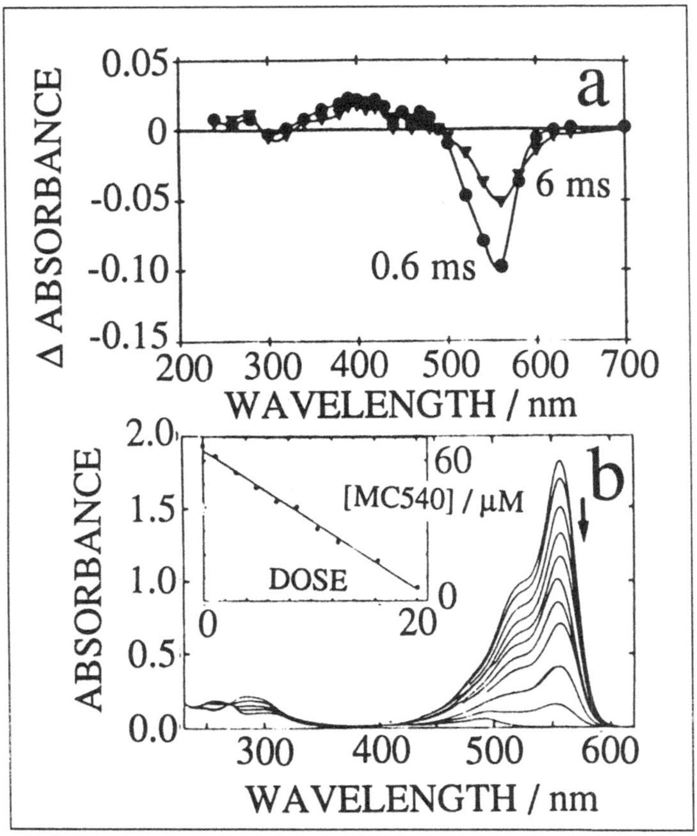

Fig. 3.23. (a) Transient differential absorption spectrum observed (●) 0.6 ms and (▼) 6 ms after pulse radiolysis of MC540 in deoxygenated aqueous propan-2-ol. (b) Absorption spectral profile following steady-state radiolysis of MC540 in deoxygenated aqueous propan-2-ol showing the gradual disappearance of dye. The insert shows the effect of accumulated radiation dose (eV / N_A) on the dye concentration that leads to the derived radiation yield of 0.29 μmol J^{-1}. J Physical Chem 1991; 95: 2415-2420.

latter species decays by way of rapid disproportionation, unless an appropriate oxidant is present, giving rise to the corresponding dianion (or a protonated version).

$$\text{MC540} + e_{aq}^{-} \rightarrow \text{MC540}^{-\cdot} \quad (9)$$

$$2\text{MC540}^{-\cdot} \rightarrow \text{MC540} + \text{MC540}^{2-} \quad (10)$$

Radiation chemical studies[3] have also shown that MC540 is readily attacked by oxidizing radicals, such as peroxyl radicals, leading to complete breakdown of the dye. It is also well known that singlet molecular oxygen and free radicals[24] of many types destroy cyanine dyes by way of adding to the polymethine bridge. There is, therefore, a rich redox chemistry available for merocyanine dyes that might have important implications for in situ chemical processes.

MECHANISMS FOR LIGHT-INDUCED CYTOTOXICITY

Under illumination, MC540 is known to kill certain enveloped viruses but to be insensitive toward a non-enveloped virus.[25] It seems likely that MC540 interacts with the lipid portion of the viral envelope and it has been argued that the sulfonate group anchors the dye close (i.e. within 6 Å) to an aqueous surface.[9] Experiments made with MC540-stained acute promyelocytic leukemic HL-60 cells were also found to be consistent with the dye locating primarily within a lipid region.[17] Thus, MC540 (20 μg/ml) was incubated with HL-60 cells (3×10^6 cells/ml) in the presence of 0.25% human serum albumin. This corresponds to a dye loading of ca. 6×10^9 molecules per cell and is typical of the concentrations used for PDT-type studies. The dye is highly fluorescent under these conditions, such that the cells are clearly visible by fluorescence microscopy. Fluorescence excitation spectra were considered to be consistent with most of the dye residing in a fairly nonpolar environment but time-resolved fluorescence studies indicated that dye was present in a distribution of sites. As such, singlet energy transfer might take place between adjacent dye molecules.

HL-60 cells are roughly spherical with 10-15 μm diameter, for which the lipid envelope constitutes approximately 25-50% of the dry weight.[26] Assuming the lipid accounts for 50% of the total volume of the cell, it can be calculated that the density of MC540 molecules present within the lipid membrane is on the order of 3×10^{12} molecules/cm^2. It has been postulated that MC540 resides within the lipid bilayers in two interchangeable orientations: parallel and perpendicular to the plane of the membrane with the parallel molecules being in equilibrium with dimers.[9] Occupancy of the parallel sites (see Fig. 3.10) is about twice that of the perpendicular sites so that dimerization of MC540 might be considerable. These dimers, which exhibit pronounced absorption bands to the red and blue of the monomer absorption band, do not fluoresce. By comparison to MC540 dispersed in neutral micelles, it has been concluded that about 30% of the total MC540 dissolved in the lipid portion of HL-60 cells at the above-mentioned loading is present in a non-fluorescent state.[17] Thus, the density of photoactive MC540 in the lipid region of each HL-60 cell is ca. 2×10^{12} molecules/cm^2 and, on average, molecules are situated ca. 40 Å apart. This spacing is sufficiently close for singlet energy transfer between dye molecules to compete with other deactivation modes for the excited state, especially with favorable orientations. In this case, reaction might occur at a site far removed from where absorption of the photon takes place.

Regardless of the viscosity or polarity of the local environment, the quantum yield for population of the triplet excited state of these MC540 molecules will not exceed 0.02 (note that laser flash photolysis studies made with MC540 incorporated into intact biological cells have shown that photoisomerization to the *cis* isomer occurs under such conditions). The inherent rate of nonradiative deactivation of the triplet state for intracellular MC540 after deoxygenation was measured to be 5×10^4 s^{-1}. The actual triplet lifetime in air-equilibrated media was found to be ca. 8 μs, indicating that molecular oxygen quenches about 70% of triplets present in the lipid membrane.[17] This quenching action might result in generation of singlet molecular oxygen, $O_2(^1\Delta_g)$, although this could not be confirmed experimentally. Under illumination with a steady photon flux of 10^{16} photons/cm^2 per minute (this value being typical of our photolysis conditions), of which approximately 30% will be absorbed by MC540, the rate of production of $O_2(^1\Delta_g)$ could approach 3×10^{10} molecules per minute irradiation per ml of solution. In terms of an individual cell, approximately 10,000 molecules of $O_2(^1\Delta_g)$ could be formed per minute illumination. These are optimistic values, assuming instant replenishment of oxygen within the lipid and further assuming quantitative formation of $O_2(^1\Delta_g)$ upon interaction between oxygen and triplet MC540.

This level of reactivity is very low and seems unlikely to be sufficient for light-induced production of $O_2(^1\Delta_g)$ to be solely responsible for cytotoxicity if it is considered that $O_2(^1\Delta_g)$ must migrate to and attack a target. It is also necessary to inquire into the fate of any $O_2(^1\Delta_g)$ so produced since many researchers appear to be convinced that $O_2(^1\Delta_g)$ peroxidation of the lipid represents the major cell-killing route.[27-30] However, much of the $O_2(^1\Delta_g)$ generated under these conditions will be formed at a site close to the aqueous phase and will be rapidly deactivated upon entering the water.[31] This crop of $O_2(^1\Delta_g)$ will not contribute significantly toward cell death. Of the remaining $O_2(^1\Delta_g)$ that stays in the lipid membrane where the diffusion length[32] is ca. 100 Å, we expect that most will react with MC540 since this is in close proximity and, relative to lipid, quenches $O_2(^1\Delta_g)$ very effectively.[17] About 5% of such encounters result in chemical modification of the dye—this being evident by the rapid bleaching of intracellular MC540 that takes place under illumination. A small fraction of lipid-bound $O_2(^1\Delta_g)$ might attack other constituents of the medium, including the lipid itself, but these tend to be relatively slow reactions that require numerous collisions before reaction takes place. It is necessary to be mindful of the short diffusion length of $O_2(^1\Delta_g)$ in a viscous hydrocarbon.[32]

Experiments relating to the effects of $O_2(^1\Delta_g)$ quenchers[30,33] or deuteration of the solvent[27,34,35] are highly conflicting and probably meaningless since few, if any, of the quencher/promoters will enter the lipid membrane where the $O_2(^1\Delta_g)$ is supposedly reacting. Similarly, claims that molecular oxygen is or is not mandatory for effective cell killing[23,35] provide no useful guidelines by which to assess likely reaction mechanisms since no real details have ever been supplied. Instead, it is our opinion that the only significant role played by $O_2(^1\Delta_g)$ in these systems is to attack and chemically modify MC540.[17] This chemical reaction[36] undoubtedly produces cytotoxic reagents possessing long diffusion lengths that are highly efficacious in killing HL-60 cells. The in situ bleaching of MC540 is not cyclic but complete conversion of dye into toxin, as indeed happens under PDT conditions, could generate up to 6×10^9 molecules of toxin per cell. This would require about one hour irradiation.

Other cytotoxicity mechanisms are possible and it is likely that processes such as light-induced electron transfer[17] and photo-isomerization[15] make a small contribution to the overall reaction. Also, since much of the dye resides in a non-photoactive (i.e. aggregated) state within the lipid membrane it is important to consider that light absorbed by these species will be rapidly converted into heat. Davila et al have considered[17] the significance of photothermal effects taking place with HL-60 cells and it is sure that such processes contribute toward cell death when high-intensity laser illumination is used. This is a cyclic process that does not consume dye and it has to be stressed that small increases in temperature are sufficient to disrupt the lipid membrane.[37,38] Such temperature changes are easily achieved with laser illumination.

So far, we have only considered the situation that it is the bulk dye that causes light-induced cytotoxicity. An alternative explanation is that a tiny fraction of the total MC540 penetrates to a critical region of the cell where it binds to some essential constituent. Under illumination, reaction with this key element causes its malfunction and thereby induces cell death. Clearly, we have no information about such a possibility. Furthermore, we have failed to identify any correlation between diffusion coefficient and efficacy for light-induced cytotoxicity observed for MC540 derivatives. Even so, we cannot rule out such possible reaction mechanisms.

It is now opportune to discuss the effects of structural modification of MC540 in light of the above-mentioned potential cytotoxicity mechanisms. The clearest structure-reactivity criterion observed with MC540 derivatives is that reported by Benniston et al.[40] These authors found an excellent correlation between cell-killing efficacy towards HL-60 cells and the partition coefficient of the dye (Fig. 3.24). Increasing the lipophilicity of the dye was matched by a substantial increase in the efficacy for light-induced cytotoxicity without there being any significant change in the photophysical properties of the dye. This effect relates to the solubility and distribution of dye inside the cell. Hydrophilic derivatives simply do not penetrate easily into the cellular membrane but prefer to remain in the outer aqueous phase. It is important to note from these studies that the variation in cell killing efficacy achieved by perturbing the lipophilicity of the dye covers more than five orders of magnitude.

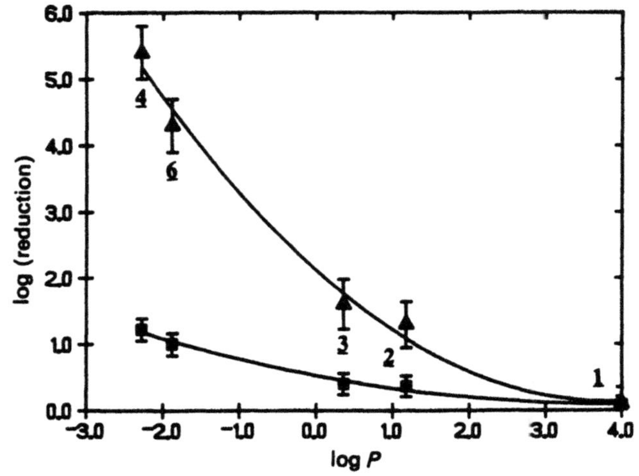

*Fig. 3.24. Correlation between the measured partition coefficient (P) and cell-killing efficacy measured after exposure to 40 J/cm² (■) and 90 J/cm² (▲) illumination at 514 nm for various merocyanine dyes. Compound labeling refers to (1) merocyanine **3**, (2) MC540, (3) merocyanine **4**, (4) merocyanine **1** and (6) merocyanine **5**. Reprinted with permission from J Chem Soc Faraday Trans 1994; 90:953-961.*

The most comprehensive structure-reactivity studies made in this area concern the elegant work reported by Günter and coworkers.[19,20] These authors described the light-induced antiviral and antileukemic properties of a wide range of MC540 derivatives. Again, it was observed that major changes in biocidal activity could be achieved by changing the structure of the dye and, in particular, incorporating selenium into the molecular backbone was found to markedly enhance the performance of the dye. Many important correlations were established by this study.[19,20] For example, it was noted that cellular and viral inactivation was curbed if the alkyl substituents on the barbiturate unit were made more lipophilic than butyl groups. This finding seems to be in excellent accord with the work of Benniston et al and probably also relates to the partition coefficient. Small changes in the length of the anchoring chain had no apparent effect on the biocidal activity. A dramatic enhancement in photodynamic efficacy was obtained by expanding the size of the benzoxazole unit, and this strategy appears to provide the most effective class of photosensitizers. Replacing sulfur with oxygen in the 2-position of the barbiturate unit decreased the photoactivity by a significant factor while replacing sulfur with selenium increased the activity. It was considered by the authors that this variation reflected changes in lipophilicity, with the more lipophilic derivatives being the more active ones. Subsequent studies with several of the compounds synthesized for this project indicated substantial changes in the photophysical properties of the dyes, especially the efficiency for production of $O_2(^1\Delta_g)$ in fluid solution.

Redmond et al have reported[22] a direct correlation between cell-killing efficacy and triplet quantum yield for a small series of merocyanine derivatives. Unfortunately, in their haste to establish such a correlation, and thereby confirm the importance of $O_2(^1\Delta_g)$ as a reaction intermediate, these authors failed to consider any other possible correlations with their data. In fact, an equally good correlation exists between cell-killing efficacy and lipophilicity of the dye. This latter correlation is extended if the results obtained by Benniston et al[21] are included (Fig. 3.25) and it seems likely that the correlation with triplet quantum yield is incidental. Certainly, there is overwhelming evidence to support the contention that the lipophilicity is of critical importance in controlling the light-induced cytotoxicity of such compounds.

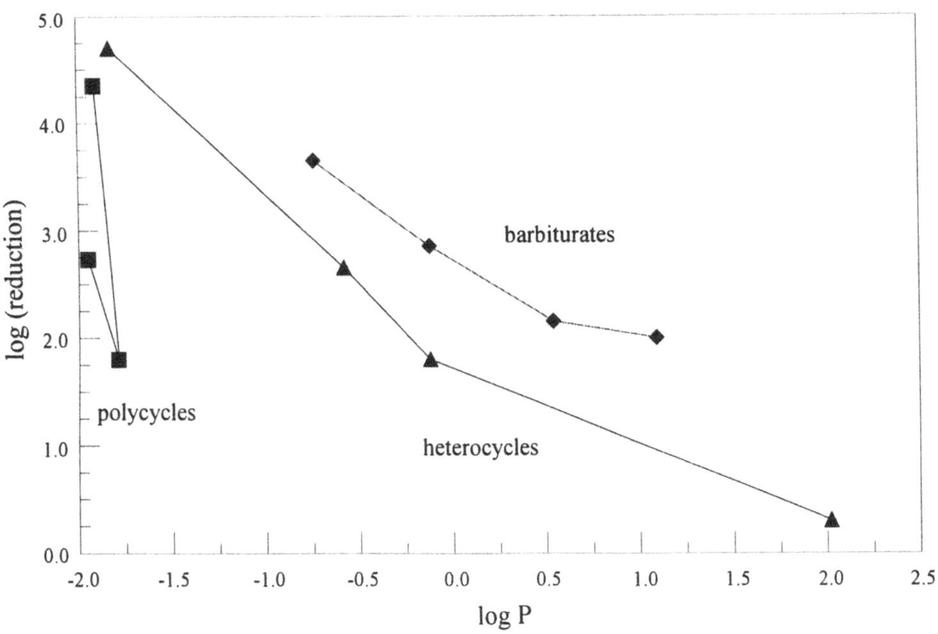

Fig. 3.25. Observed correlation between the efficacy for light-induced cytotoxicity towards HL-60 leukemia cells (expressed as log reduction in cell viability) and the partition coefficient. The compounds are classified according to the nature of the substituent: "barbiturates" refer to merocyanines 2, 13, 14 and 15, "heterocycles" refer to MC540 and merocyanines 2, 11 and 12, and "polycycles" refer to merocyanines 5, 6 and 10. Photophysical data for these compounds are given in the various tables.

Overall, it is apparent that the biocidal activity of MC540 can be modulated by synthetic methodology. Most attempts reported to date have been concerned with trying to improve the triplet quantum yield in an effort to increase the ability of the dye to photosensitize production of $O_2(^1\Delta_g)$ or with changing the lipophilicity of the dye. The most effective new generation photosensitizers still suffer from the same problem encountered with MC540 in that they accumulate in the lipid envelope of leukemic cells and are rapidly bleached under illumination. Following from the original studies of Günter et al,[19,20] it is well established that incorporating a selenium atom into the molecular skeleton, especially in the barbiturate subunit, markedly improves the performance of the dye. Under such conditions, the triplet quantum yield is much higher than that found for MC540 (see Table 3.5) while the dye is much more lipophilic—both factors contributing to its enhanced performance.

MOLECULAR RECOGNITION PATTERNS

The one property that distinguishes MC540 from many other potential PDT photosensitizers, and that which makes the compound special, concerns its apparent preferential affinity for leukemic and certain other types of neoplastic cells, even in the presence of mature healthy cells.[25] The mechanism of this affinity appears to be, at least in part, due to the less-ordered state of organization of lipids in the neoplastic cell membranes.[39] Apparently this state can be induced by activation of cells with appropriate stimuli, transformation or viral infections. In any event, this is a remarkable feat of molecular recognition that, once optimized by further synthetic chemistry, holds genuine promise for effecting a means for the early detection and possible therapeutic treatment of leukemia. In fact, it can be argued that the single most important aspect of this work relates to the identification of improved methods for detection of leukemia during the earliest stages of illness, especially for those patients undergoing chemotherapy. It is essential, therefore, that we address the issues which by themselves allow recognition of leukemic cells with merocyanine dyes.

Although still very much at a preliminary stage,[18] we have started to explore systematically the structural attributes of MC540 with a view to identifying the key recognition elements (Structure 3.13). From this perspective, the molecule can be subdivided

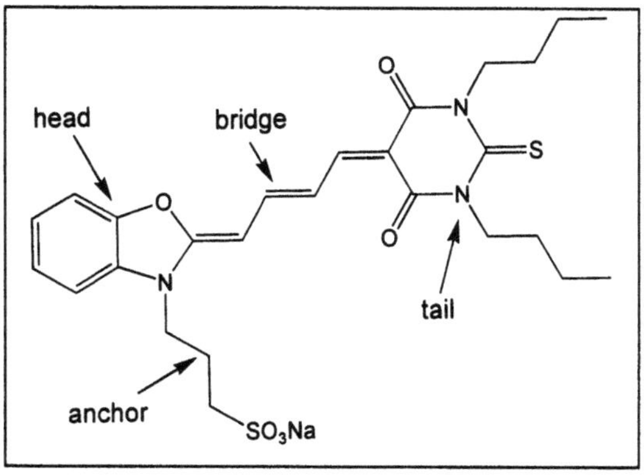

Structure 3.13. Structural attributes of MC540.

into four parts namely, head, tail, anchor and polymethine bridge. These various units can be varied independently and the resultant structures tested for their ability to selectively recognize leukemic cells in the presence of excess (e.g. 100-fold) normal cells. Remembering that most of the MC540 derivatives synthesized to date are highly fluorescent when incorporated into biological cells, it follows that stained cells (leukemic or healthy) can be monitored by flow cytometry with fluorescence detection. Trial experiments show that the amount of exposure to illumination under such conditions is insufficient to bleach the dye such that reliable cell counts can be achieved in this way at quite low loadings of dye.

The first important point to emerge from these studies is that the presence of the sulfonate residue is mandatory for cell recognition and assimilation. Without this water-solubilizing group (e.g. replacing MC540 with merocyanine **1**) the dye is readily incorporated into intact cells, being more easily taken up than is MC540, and very photoactive once inside the cell membrane. This compound is extremely effective as a photosensitizer for the light-induced inactivation of the Herpes simplex virus but it displays no preference for selective uptake by leukemic cells relative to healthy cells.

Replacing the sulfonic acid group with a carboxylic acid residue restores the basic recognition pattern but does not improve it. Similarly, the length of the alkyl chain on the anchor moiety does not seem to be important with respect to recognition of neoplastic cells, provided it is at least three carbon atoms long. The possibility of using branched chains has not yet been explored. Finally, the nature of the counter cation seems to afford no effect on the recognition process. We may surmise, therefore, that a propyl sulfonate chain should be retained in the final structure.

We have seen that the thiobarbiturate unit can be easily modified so as to modulate the solubility and partition coefficient. There is, of course, a marked correlation between light-induced cell killing efficacy and the partition coefficient of the dye as described above. The nature of the alkyl chains attached to the amido nitrogen atoms carry some recognition elements but this feature is somewhat obscured by the corresponding effect on the total uptake of dye. That is to say, the alkyl chains determine, at least to a large degree, the amount of dye that can be assimilated into biological cells and the rate of uptake. Longer chains give higher in situ concentrations but the rate of uptake reaches a maximum for hexyl chains. The longer chain analogues show slightly more preference for selective uptake by leukemic cells but the overall benefit does not exceed a factor of four-fold, as found with hexadecyl chains.

The corresponding bis-oxonol derivatives,[40] comprising two thiobarbiturate units linked via the usual polymethine bridge (Structure 3.14), are potent photosensitizers for light-induced destruction of HL-60 leukemic cells. They possess no ability to assimilate into neoplastic cells rather than healthy cells, even though they are equipped with the appropriate thiobarbiturate units and the polymethine bridge. It seems likely, therefore, that recognition of leukemic cells demands the presence of the benzoxazole head group.

The length of the polymethine bridge can be varied,[1] at the cost of synthetic simplicity. Changing the number of methine groups in the bridge has a profound effect on the properties of the dye, especially the absorption maximum, and causes major

Structure 3.14. Structures of the bis-oxonols.

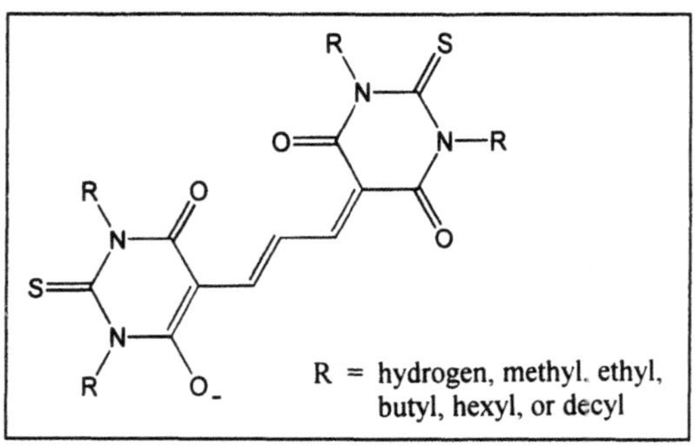

changes in the rate of photoisomerization. In no case, however, does this strategy result in a substantially enhanced triplet quantum yield. We are unaware of any attempts to correlate the length of the polymethine bridge with the ability of the dye to recognize leukemic cells. It seems reasonable, given our present state of knowledge, to retain the butadienyl chain, at least until more information becomes available.

Finally, the nature of the head group has been found to exert a pronounced influence on the ability of the dye to recognize and penetrate into infected cells. Extending the benzoxazole head group by fusing on an extra benzene ring, giving rise to the three isomeric naphthoxazole derivatives, has a marked effect on the recognition pattern. Indeed, using a very simple assaying method in which dye is mixed separately with a fixed number (i.e. 2×10^6 cells/ml) of leukemic and healthy cells, it has been possible to estimate a crude measure of the cellular recognition properties of these merocyanine dyes. Under these predetermined conditions, the relative assimilation of dye into neoplastic versus normal cells, as monitored by polarized fluorescence microscopy which detects only assimilated dye, can be expressed in the following form:

$$R = N_L/N_N \tag{11}$$

Here, N_L and N_N, respectively, refer to the number of leukemic and normal cells labeled with a particular fluorescent dye. Table 3.6 lists the results of this study. It seems clear that a substantial improvement in the recognition properties of such merocyanine dyes can be obtained by varying the nature of the head group. It appears that a "blunt head" is better than a "sharp head" in attaining high levels of cellular specificity. This realization might be consistent with the rate limiting step being penetration of a lipid membrane, since the origin of the selectivity is of a kinetic nature. There is no exchange of dye from leukemic to normal cells upon diluting the suspension with healthy cells. However, it should be stressed that additional experiments are urgently needed to address the issue of whether or not the dye shows preferential recognition of leukemic cells when these are in the presence of excess normal cells.

It should be noted, however, that replacing MC540 with the somewhat related kryptocyanine derivative[41] (Structure 3.15) loses all selective recognition for leukemic cells. The positively-charged

Table 3.6. Quantitative assessment of the ability of merocyanine dyes to assimilate into leukemic cells in preference to normal cells (The conditions were not optimized with respect to the amount of serum protein used as carrier and it is likely that consistently higher selectivity factors could be attained by careful control of the ancillary medium.)

Merocyanine Dye	Selectivity Factor R
MC540	27
1	8
2	33
4	65
5	180
6	35
10	115

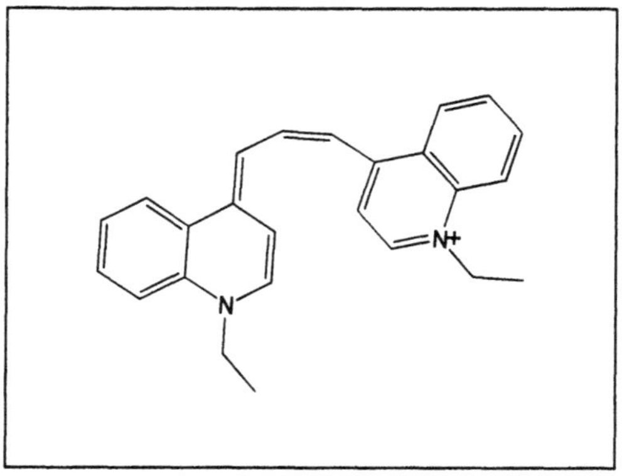

Structure 3.15. Structure of kryptocyanine.

kryptocyanine tends to localize in the mitochondrial membrane where it exerts a useful photodynamic effect, possibly by blocking the transport of quinone-bearing enzymatic functions. It does not penetrate easily into intact biological cells nor does it intercalate into DNA. Moreover, it does not distinguish between neoplastic and healthy cells.

REFERENCES

1. Hamer FM. The Cyanine Dyes and Related Compounds. New York: Wiley Interscience, 1964:706-42.
2. Harriman A, Shoute LCT, Neta P. Radiation chemistry of cyanine dyes: oxidation and reduction of merocyanine 540. J Phys Chem 1991; 95:2415-20.

3. Benniston AC, Harriman A, Gulliya KS. Photophysical properties of Merocyanine 540 derivatives. J Chem Soc, Faraday Trans 1994; 90:953-61.
4. Gordon AJ, Ford RA. The Chemist's Companion. Chichester: Wiley-Interscience, 1972:184.
5. Kushner KM, Smith CP. Resonance and polarity in the molecules of three colored compounds. J Am Chem Soc 1949; 71:1401-40.
6. Gulliya KS, Davila J, Harriman A. The mechanism of LDL-mediated increased uptake of Merocyanine 540 by HL-60 cells. The Cancer J 1990; 3:360-65.
7. Gulliya KS, Mathews JL, Fay JW, Dowben RM. Increased survival of normal cells during laser photodynamic therapy; implications for ex-vivo autologous bone marrow purging. Life Sci 1988; 42:2651-6.
8. Gulliya KS, Pervaiz S. Elimination of clonogenic tumor cells from HL-60, Daudi and U-937 cell lines by laser photoradiation therapy; implications for autologous bone marrow purging. Blood 1989; 73:1059-65.
9. Dragsten PR, Webb WW. Mechanism of the membrane potential sensitivity of the fluorescent membrane probe Merocyanine 540. Biochemistry 1978; 17:5228-40.
10. Dixit NS, Mackay RA. Absorption and emission characteristics of Merocyanine 540 in microemulsions. J Am Chem Soc 1983; 105:2928-29.
11. Aramendia PH, Krieg M, Nitsch C, Bittersman E, Braslavsky SE. The photophysics of Merocyanine 540: A comparative study in ethanol and in liposomes. Photochem Photobiol 1988; 48:187-94.
12. Aramendia PH, Duchowicz R, Schaffardi L, Tocho JO. Photophysical characterization of a photochromic system; The case of Merocyanine 540. J Phys Chem 1990; 94: 1389-92.
13. Hoebeke M, Piette J, Van der Vorst A. Viscosity-dependent isomerization and fluorescence yields of Merocyanine 540. J Photochem Photobiol, B Biol 1990; 4:273-82.
14. Hoebeke M, Seret A, Piette J, Van der Vorst A. Singlet oxygen production and photoisomerization;competitive processes for Merocyanine 540 irradiated with visible light. J Photochem Photobiol, B Biol 1988; 1:437-46.
15. Davila J, Gulliya KS, Harriman A. Inactivation of tumours and viruses via efficient photoisomerization. J Chem Soc, Chem Commun 1989; 1215-16.
16. Harriman A. Photoisomerization dynamics of merocyanine dyes in solution. J Photochem Photobiol, A Chem 1992; 65:79-93.
17. Davila J, Harriman A, Gulliya KS. Photochemistry of Merocyanine 540: The mechanism of chemotherapeutic activity with cyanine dyes. Photochem Photobiol 1991; 53:1-11.
18. Benniston AC, Harriman A. To be published.
19. Günter WHH, Searle R, Sieber F. Structure-activity relationships in the antiviral and antileukemic photoproperties of Merocyanine 540. Seminars in Hematology 1992; 29:88-94.

20. Günter WHH, Searle R, Sieber F. Photosensitizing merocyanine dyes based on selenobarbituric acid. Phosphorus, Sulfur, and Silicon 1992; 67:417.
21. Benniston AC, Harriman A, Gulliya KS. To be published.
22. Redmond RW, Srichai MB, Bilitz JM, Schlomer DD, Krieg M. Merocyanine dyes: Effect of structural modifications on photophyical properties and biological activity. Photochem Photobiol 1994; 60:348-55.
23. Feix JB, Kalyanaraman B. An electron spin resonance study of Merocyanine 540-mediated type I reactions in liposomes. Photochem Photobiol 1991; 53:39-45.
24. Byers GW, Gross S, Henriches PM. Direct and sensitized photooxidation of cyanine dyes. Photochem Photobiol 1976; 23:37-43.
25. Sieber F. Merocyanine 540. Photochem Photobiol 1987; 46: 1035-42.
26. O'Neil CH. Isolation and properties of the cell surface membrane of Amoeba Proteus. Expt Cell Res 1964; 35: 477-96.
27. Kalyanaraman B, Feix JB, Sieber F, Thomas JP, Girotti AW. Photodynamic action of Merocyanine 540 on artificial and natural cell membranes: involvement of singlet molecular oxygen. Proc Natl Acad Sci 1987; 84:2999-3003.
28. Feix JB, Kalyanaraman B, Chignell CF, Hall RD. Direct observation of singlet oxygen production by merocyanine 540 associated with phosphatidylcholine liposomes. J. Biol. Chem. 1988; 263:17247-50.
29. O'Brien JM, Montgomery RR, Burns WH, Gaffney DK, Sieber F. Evaluation of Merocyanine 540-sensitized photoirradiation as a means to inactivate enveloped viruses in blood products. J Lab Clin Med 1990; 116:439-47.
30. Gaffney DK, O'Brien JM, Sieber F. Modulation by thiols of the Merocyanine 540-sensitized photolysis of leukemia cells, red cells, and herpes simplex virus type I. Photochem Photobiol 1991; 53:85-92.
31. Rodgers MAJ, Snowden PT. Lifetime of $O_2(^1\Delta_g)$ in liquid water as determined by time-resolved infra-red luminescence measurements. J Am Chem Soc 1982; 104:5541-43.
32. Moan J. On the diffusion length of singlet oxygen in cells and tissue. J Photochem Photobiol, B Biol 1990; 6: 343-44.
33. Gulliya KS, Mathews JL, Fay JW, Dowben RM. Effect of free radical quenchers on the dye-mediated laser light induced photosensitization of leukemic cells. Proc SPIE 1987; 847: 163-65.
34. Gaffney DK, Schober SL, Sieber F. Merocyanine 540-sensitized photoinactivation of leukemic cells: role of oxygen and effects on plasma membrane integrity and mitochondrial respiration. Exp Hematol 1990; 18:23-26.

35. O'Brien JM, Siebe F. Merocyanine 540-sensitized photoinactivation of enveloped viruses and its application in the sterilization of blood products. In: Gorin NC, Douay L, eds. Experimental Hematology Today. New York: Springer, 1989:26-30.
36. Franck B, Schneider U. Photooxidation products of merocyanine 540 formed under preactivation conditions for tumor therapy. Photochem Photobiol 1992; 56: 271-76.
37. Nagle JF. Theory of biomembrane phase transitions. J Chem Phys 1973; 58:252-64.
38. Srinivasan KR, Kay RL, Nagle JF. The pressure dependence of lipid bilayer phase transition. Biochemistry 1974; 13:3494-96.
39. McEvoy L, Schlegel RA, Williamson P et al. Merocyanine 540 as flow cytometric probe of membrane lipid organization in leukocytes. J Leukocyte Biol 1988; 44:337-44.
40. Benniston AC, Harriman A. Photoinduced and thermal isomerization processes for bis-oxonols: Rotor volume, stereochemical and viscosity effects. J Chem Soc, Faraday Trans 1994; 90: 2627-34.
41. Harriman A, Luengo G, Gulliya KS. In vitro photodynamic activity of kryptocyanine. Photochem Photobiol 1990; 52:735-40.

CHAPTER 4

Preclinical Studies of Preactivated Merocyanine 540 and Merodantoin

It is apparent from the discussion in the previous chapters that photoproducts in pMC540 display a significant toxicity against cultured tumor cells and enveloped viruses but are only minimally cytotoxic to normal cells. A question of obvious significance is whether these findings from in vitro studies have any relevance to cancer or viral infections in humans. In this chapter, we shall examine the data obtained from studies utilizing in vivo models that support further development of these compounds for ultimate clinical use.

BACKGROUND

The transition from in vitro experiments to in vivo experiments requires the use of animal models. Models by definition are a simulation, generally in miniature or a copy of something that shows or mimics either structure and/or function, so that the model is no different from the thing being modeled except, perhaps in size. For human cancer, unfortunately there are no satisfactory models. This may be in part due to the heterogeneity of human cancers as well as humans themselves. A widely different response of tumors to chemotherapy, ranging from no response to complete response, exemplifies the heterogeneity of tumors. This problem is further compounded by the diverse responses of individuals, both human

Novel Chemotherapeutic Agents: Preactivation in the Treatment of Cancer and AIDS, by K. S. Gulliya.

and animal to the chemotherapeutic agents used. It has been demonstrated that the growth kinetics and drug responses of tumors obtained from the same donor differ significantly in response to identical treatments. Even with these difficulties, in vivo tumor models in general do provide important useful information that otherwise could not be obtained. Thus, in vivo models are an indispensable part of new drug development.

It is also noteworthy, however, that although almost all currently used antitumor drugs were shown to have antitumor activity in animal models of one type or another, there are few clinically effective drugs that did not produce any effect in most commonly used animal models employing L1210, P388, B16 and Lewis lung tumors. Examples of such drugs are busulfan and hexamethylmelamine (shown to be effective against Walker 256 carcinosarcoma and Dunning leukemia of rats), L-asparaginase (effective in tumors lacking L-asparagine synthetase), and hormones (used because of the known hormonal dependence of certain tumors). Therefore, lack of response in a given tumor model to a new drug in question should be viewed with caution.

One of the most unfortunate side effects and hazards of chemotherapy is the death of a patient. Death occurs, in part, because of the variable response of the patients to the same dose of drug. Some patients will experience only a mild side effect whereas others will suffer serious toxicity. But the main reason for serious side effects and death is the very narrow therapeutic window of the currently available anticancer drugs. Taken together, these factors alone reduce the margin of error considerably. New drugs are developed and used with the expectation that they will yield better results in terms of their efficacy and lack of systemic toxicity. The basic aim of toxicological studies, therefore, is to determine the degree and kind of harmful effect before a drug is considered safe for therapeutic purposes in humans. According to federal government regulations, toxicological studies should involve at least three animal species, of which one should be a nonrodent. Evaluation of a new drug in animal species is usually made by the determination of dose responses, absorption of the drug, biodistribution, metabolism, half life of plasma clearance, excretion; site and mechanism of action; activity of degradation products of the drug, acute, subacute, or chronic toxicity and allergic reactions. Other toxicity studies such as teratogenic and carcinogenic properties of the test drug are also determined. Biological activity of the drug should always be tested in animals before human trials are initiated as these tests provide fairly reliable evidence of the therapeutic values and safety of the drug. Although the predictive value of data from animals and their interpretation with regard to human application is far from absolute, the pharmacological actions of the drug are, by and large, similar to those in humans. However, toxicological studies in animals pose other problems, for example, variations due to species or strain differences and translation of information from healthy animals under controlled conditions to pathological conditions in human beings. The ideal species for toxicity studies should possess the following criteria: 1) under 1 kilogram in weight; 2) easy to bleed and large enough to supply a reasonable amount of blood; 3) easy to breed and maintain in the laboratory; 4) easy to handle and to administer drugs by various routes; 5) should have short life span; 6) physiology should approximate that of humans.

The weight of the experimental animal is important because during early stages of drug development, only small quantities may be available. The choice of species is also important. A completely vegetarian species, for example, may not be useful because of the differences in the microflora of the intestine, which may affect drug metabolism. Among the various species of animals used in toxicological studies, mice, rats, dogs, pigs and nonhuman primates are most common.

Thus, toxicological studies are serious, sizable and perhaps one of the most important undertakings in drug development. In my experience (hind sight), detailed toxicological studies should be contracted out to experienced contract research organizations. This is very important if one wants to obtain data that will be useful for supporting an IND application. The process is expensive but probably not as much when one considers the lost time, resources and cost of learning curve, etc. Naturally, availability of sizable funds is usually the decisive factor here.

ABOUT THE DRUG DOSE

Before proceeding further with the description of the toxicological studies of pMC540, it is important (to make a point) to narrate a recent incident that has occurred over and over again during the past 10 years. In a phone conversation, a scientist from a major pharmaceutical company, responsible for evaluating new chemotherapeutic agents for potential licensing and development, told me that, "our scientific group thinks that the dose of your compound appears to be high and we are not used to seeing such high doses for chemotherapeutic agents." Although quite disturbed by the erroneous yet entrenched misconception in the field of drug development, I calmly explained my position on the subject.

Here is the point I made. The main goal of cancer therapy or for that matter therapy for any disease is 1) to kill the cancer and 2) spare the host. The key here is point number 2, i.e. spare the host, otherwise all that is required to do is to fetch a bottle of bleach from the nearest grocery store and use it. I guarantee that it will destroy all malignancies. But there is one major problem; it will kill the host as well. Thus, sparing the host is the key issue in drug development and the quantity of the drug used to achieve this goal is at best irrelevant. Therefore, apprehension in using or outright rejection of drugs that are effective at so-called high doses is based on tradition (perhaps resulting from the experience of using bluntly toxic materials for cancer therapy) and not on scientific reason. Therefore, I cannot stress this point strongly enough to all scientists and clinicians; look at the therapeutic window of the new agent and not the quantity (dose) of the drug. I wonder how many perfectly good therapeutic agents have been rejected because of this entrenched misconception!

TOXICITY, PLASMA CLEARANCE AND BIODISTRIBUTION OF pMC540

In the following, a discussion of data from experiments performed to assess the toxicity of preactivated merocyanine 540 is followed by its anticancer and antiviral activity in mice, cat and primate models.

In Vivo Toxicity of Preactivated Merocyanine 540

In preliminary studies, a limited number of toxicological tests of preactivated merocyanine 540 were performed in mice and pigs. In vivo toxicity and biodistribution studies were among the first set of in vivo experiments that were carried out. These toxicity studies revealed that pMC540 was significantly less toxic than the unactivated MC540 when injected into DBA/2 mice. For example, the lethal intravenous dose of pMC540 in mice was 240 mg/kg as compared to 40 mg/kg for nonactivated MC540. Intraperitoneal injection of pMC540 at doses of 370 mg/kg were lethal. Repeat dose experiments show that mice tolerated a cumulative dose of 400 mg/kg without any observable signs of toxicity.[1]

PLASMA CLEARANCE

To determine the nature of plasma clearance 50 μCi (50 μg) of ^{3}H-pMC540 was injected into DBA/2 mice. Blood samples collected at indicated time points were diluted with phosphate buffered saline (pH 7.4) and centrifuged at 1500 g for 10 minutes to remove the pelleted cellular components. An aliquot from the supernatant was taken in 10 ml of scintillation cocktail, and radioactivity was determined. Radioactive counts were converted to ng/mL of ^{3}H-pMC540 from the average DPM obtained from 50 μCi. Data from these studies show that as much as 70% of the injected radiolabeled pMC540 was excreted within 6 hours of injection and only less than 2% of the radioactivity remained in the animal body after one week. The plasma half-life of pMC540 in mice (Fig. 4.1) was calculated to be approximately 23 hours.[1] The extent of drug absorption is known to depend on surface area, blood flow, solubility of the drug and its lipophilic and hydrophilic properties. The rapid clearance of pMC540 indicates that the lipophilic nature of native MC540 was rendered more hydrophilic upon preactivation.

BIODISTRIBUTION

Studies of the distribution of pMC540 in various organs and tissues suggest that none of the major organs showed preferential accumulation of radioactive pMC540 and brain, liver and kidneys constituted the main organs accounting for the unexcreted activity (Table 4.1). Surprisingly over 48% of the radioactivity was recovered from brain after 6 hours of injection. While these results were encouraging and suggestive of further investigation, they did not prove that pMC540 or its active metabolite actually accumulate in the brain. At the time these studies were conducted one of the unresolved problems was that pMC540 could not be concentrated by freeze drying method as this procedure resulted in a significant loss in cytotoxic activity. As a result, high drug doses could not be given to large animals such as dogs and pigs due to high volume. Additionally, in view of our limited capacity to produce large quantities of preactivated material at the time, only small doses of pMC540 were used in the studies involving blood chemistry profiles.

For the studies of blood chemistry, pigs were injected with escalating (2, 3 and 5 mg/kg) doses of pMC540 through an indwelling surgical catheter. Analysis of blood samples drawn every 24 hours for a period of 7 days did not reveal any abnormality in terms of serum electrolytes, renal function, hepatic function or cardiac enzymes (Tables 4.2 and 4.3). Transient rise in creatinine phosphokinase were attributable to intramuscular injections of valium used to restrain the animal prior to pMC540 injection.

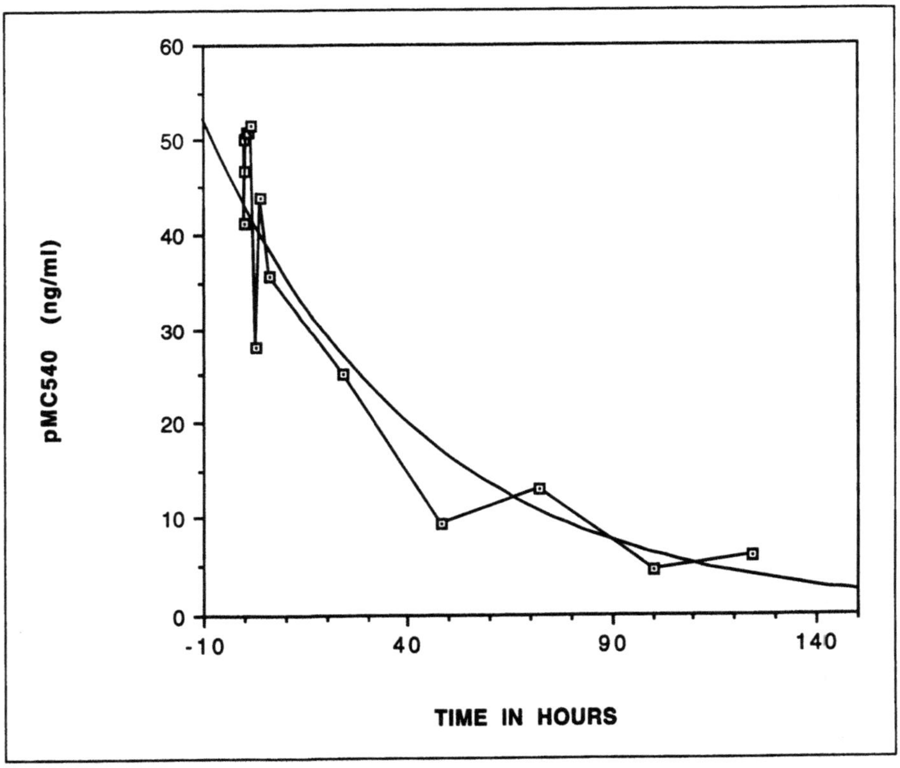

Fig. 4.1. Plasma clearance of p-^{3}H-MC540 was determined by an intraperitoneal injection of 50 μCi (50 μg) into DBA/2 mice. Blood samples were obtained at various time points. These samples were diluted with PBS (pH 7.4) and centrifuged at 1500 g for 10 minutes to pellet the cellular component. An aliquot from the supernatant was taken in 10 ml of scintillation cocktail, and radioactivity was counted using a Beckman Scintillation Counter, Model LS 1701. Radioactive counts were converted to ng/ml of p-^{3}H-MC540 from the average DPM obtained from 50 μCi. Reprinted with permission from Cancer Chemother Pharma 1993; 31:467-474.

Test of liver function which constitutes one of the most important assays, did not reveal an elevation of serum bilirubin which would be indicative of clinical jaundice. Similarly functional and mechanical damage to liver indicated by the elevation of alkaline phosphatase, which hydrolyzes phosphate ester in drug induced cholelithiasis, was not observed. Abnormalities, as determined by CBC analysis and blood-coagulation profiles were not observed as all values were within normal range. Similar results were obtained when a dog was injected with a single dose (20 mg/kg) of pMC540 and followed for a period of 30 days. Serum transaminase (AST and ALT) activity, which is elevated in hepatocellular damage caused by chemicals or toxins[2], was elevated in the dog receiving 20 mg/kg of pMC540 without any clinical signs of hepatotoxicity. Therefore, a more sensitive assay indicative of hepatotoxicity was conducted by determining the serum levels of GGT.[3] In the dog the levels of GGT remained well below the normal limits for the duration of the study, indicating that hepatocellular damage was not occurring and elevation in AST and ALT levels may be due to some nonspecific phenomenon. Serum levels of albumin also remained unchanged (albumin levels usually decrease in hepatocellular damage) further supporting our

Table 4.1. Percent distribution of ^{3}H-pMC540*

Samples	Percent of Radioactivity Injected 2 hours	4 hours	6 hours	24 hours	48 hours	96 hours	1 week
Liver	0.09	0.12	4.35	3.59	0.86	0.21	0.14
Kidney	0.07	0.06	4.49	2.64	1.19	0.31	0.21
Spleen	0.03	0.01	1.37	1.51	0.34	0.21	0.17
Heart	0.01	0.00	1.59	1.69	0.74	0.34	0.24
Brain	0.07	0.06	5.35	6.67	0.31	0.69	0.39
Lungs	0.02	0.01	1.06	0.94	0.97	0.81	0.34
Urine	ND	47.00	42.00	3.10	0.59	0.09	0.05
Feces	ND	33.00	28.00	2.74	0.67	0.11	0.06
Others	ND	19.71	11.79	7.11	15.31	1.27	0.28

* Tritium labeled preactivated merocyanine 540
ND = not determined
Data shown are mean of four separate sets of experiments consisting of 2 or 3 animals per group. The radioactivity values in urine and feces, accounting for approximately 70%, are not reflected in the amount of radioactivity recovered subsequent to six-hour time points. Reprinted with permission from Cancer Chemother Pharma 1993; 31:467-474.

conclusion. Additional support for this conclusion was provided by the studies of the coagulation profile. These data show that prothrombin time was unchanged, indicating normal activities of prothrombin, fibrinogen and factors V, VII, X, all of which are synthesized by the liver. Similarly, partial prothromboplastin time

Table 4.2. In vivo toxicity of pMC540* in pigs

Laboratory Test	Baseline	Day 0 2 mg/kg Injection	Day 1	Day 3 3 mg/kg Injection	Day 5	Day 7 5 mg/kg Injection	Day 15	Day 30
SMAC-28								
Glucose	96.0	111.0	105.0	108.0	139.0	130.0	128.0	114.0
Sodium	139.0	143.0	142.0	147.0	143.0	142.0	144.0	140.0
Potassium	3.7	3.8	4.1	4.4	4.5	4.0	4.3	3.8
Chloride	100.0	103.0	103.0	105.0	100.0	101.0	100.0	105.0
CO_2	30.0	23.0	24.0	24.0	23.0	24.0	23.0	30.0
Anion Gap	9.0	17.0	15.0	18.0	20.0	17.0	19.0	11.0
BUN	7.0	16.0	14.0	15.0	12.0	10.0	13.0	8.0
Creatinine	1.0	1.2	1.0	1.1	1.3	1.0	1.1	1.0
BUN/Creatinine	7.0	13.0	14.0	13.0	9.0	10.0	9.0	8.0
Cholesterol, Total	83.0	106.0	106.0	92.0	95.0	88.0	96.0	86.0
Triglycerides	16.0	28.0	53.0	31.0	51.0	36.0	50.0	30.0
LDL-Cholesterol	35.0	56.0	51.0	41.0	40.0	36.0	40.0	34.0
VLDL-Cholesterol	3.0	5.0	10.0	6.0	10.0	7.0	9.0	6.0
Uric Acid	0.4	0.3	0.2	0.1	0.3	0.1	0.1	0.2
Phosphorus	6.8	6.3	7.4	7.5	8.2	6.9	8.0	6.9
Calcium	9.5	10.0	9.7	9.1	9.9	9.5	9.5	9.4
Total Protein	6.3	7.4	6.9	6.5	6.9	6.5	6.9	6.4
Albumin	3.2	3.7	3.5	3.3	3.5	3.2	3.5	3.3
Globulin	3.1	3.7	3.4	3.2	3.4	3.3	3.7	3.2
A/G Ratio	1.0	1.0	1.0	1.0	1.0	1.0	1.0	1.0
Bilirubin, Total	0.1	0.1	0.1	0.1	0.1	0.2	0.1	0.2
Bilirubin, Direct	0.0	0.0	0.0	0.0	0.0	0.1	0.0	0.1
Alkaline Phosphatase	131.0	140.0	131.0	155.0	159.0	138.0	146.0	134.0
GGT	50.0	47.0	50.0	46.0	51.0	49.0	50.0	49.0
AST (SGOT)	27.0	28.0	38.0	40.0	20.0	27.0	29.0	28.0
ALT (SGPT)	36.0	37.0	43.0	39.0	38.0	39.0	39.0	37.0
LDH	467.0	493.0	440.0	451.0	472.0	354.0	384.0	450.0
CPK	670.0	1677.0	2235.0	422.0	313.0	689.0	386.0	464.0
Iron	101.0	131.0	167.0	96.0	41.0	104.0	110.0	105.0

*Preactivated merocyanine 540. Reprinted with permission from Cancer Chemother Pharma 1993; 31:467-474.

remained unchanged, indicating normal activities of prothrombin, fibrinogen, and factors V, VII, IX and XI and that pMC540 did not cause endothelial damage and is nonthrombogenic. Similar results were obtained from the analysis of blood samples from pMC540 treated dogs.

While the data presented indicates that pMC540 was very easily tolerated at doses tested in mice, pigs and dogs, it is important to note that due to different routes of drug injections, bioavailability and absorption characteristics in mice (i.p.) and in pigs and dogs (i.v.), an interspecies comparison of this data cannot be made.

PRECLINICAL ANTIVIRAL ACTIVITY OF pMC540

EFFECT OF pMC540 IN THE TREATMENT OF FELINE IMMUNODEFICIENCY VIRUS

In a discussion with Dr. Bruce Wiggs, chairman of animal care and use committee, regarding the in vitro and in vivo observations made with pMC540, we learned that some of his patients

Table 4.3. In vivo toxicity of pMC540* in pigs

Laboratory Test	Baseline	Day 0 2 mg/kg Injection	Day 1	Day 3 3 mg/kg Injection	Day 5	Day 7 5 mg/kg Injection	Day 15	Day 30
CBC w/Differential								
Platelet Count								
WBC	13.0	16.1	16.7	16.1	22.3	18.7	15.1	14.3
RBC	6.3	7.4	6.9	7.3	6.8	6.1	6.3	6.4
Hemoglobin	11.2	13.3	12.2	11.9	12.0	10.8	11.1	11.2
Hematocrit	33.0	39.6	36.5	37.8	36.5	33.0	34.0	33.0
MCV	53.0	53.0	53.0	54.0	54.0	55.0	54.0	53.0
MCH	17.9	17.9	17.8	17.7	17.8	17.9	17.9	17.9
MCHC	33.9	33.6	33.4	34.1	32.9	32.7	33.9	33.8
RDW	19.6	19.9	19.6	19.7	21.8	21.0	20.0	20.0
Platelet Count	310.0	305.0	275.0	296.0	397.0	273.0	305.0	310.0
MPV	9.2	10.9	10.7	10.8	9.1	8.8	9.4	9.3
Lymphocytes %	66.5	52.0	49.0	54.0	38.0	65.0	66.0	67.0
Monocytes %	8.9	15.0	04.0	10.0	10.0	3.0	9.0	10.0
Granulocytes %	24.6	33.0	47.0	36.0	52.0	32.0	25.0	23.0

*Preactivated merocyanine 540. Reprinted with permission from Cancer Chemother Pharma 1993; 31:467-474.

(cats), suffering from lymphocytic plasmacytic stomatitis, associated with feline leukemia virus (FeLV) and feline immunodeficiency virus (FIV), failed to respond to all conventional treatments given to them. Therefore, as a last resort, with owners' permission, Dr. Wiggs treated two cats with pMC540. Subsequent literature survey revealed that cats infected with FIV were a desirable model for human immunodeficiency virus.[4] FIV, a lentivirus from the retrovirus group, is similar to HIV and equinine infectious anemia (EIA). Feline leukemia virus is type-C oncornavirus of the retrovirus group. Although the causative agent of lymphocytic-plasmacytic stomatitis is unknown, the disease is commonly seen in association with FIV and FeLV. The following is a brief description of the case history of cats and their response to the pMC540 treatment.

The first cat subjected to pMC540 treatment was a neutered male of unknown age (adopted as a stray). This cat. weighing 8.9 pounds, had a history of gradual weight loss and severe chronic stomatitis. The cat had received treatments which included a complete dental prophylaxis, extraction of all molar and premolar teeth (due to extensive stomatitis and development of resorptive cervical line lesions) and a number of antibiotics. None of these treatments produced improvements lasting more than a few weeks. However, anti-inflammatory corticosteroids were not given, because a housemate was positive for FIV. Following these failed attempts at treatment, the animal was presented again for re-evaluation. At this time, the animal's mouth odor was so strong that it could be easily detected from a distance of approximately 10-15 feet. Gingival tissues were highly inflamed, with a mucoid, brown threadlike saliva and spontaneous bleeding of the gums. Periodontal disease was present, with one additional small resorptive lesion on the right mandibular cuspid.

To establish baseline control values, pre-treatment blood work including CBC, SMA, FIP, FIA, FIV and FeLV were performed. Cultures and biopsies of the gum tissues were submitted to the laboratory included calcivirus testing. In house Cite®, Combo™ FIV/FeLV tests (IDEXX Labs, Inc., Westbrook, Maine) were also performed. Laboratory and in house tests revealed that the animal was positive for FIV and FeLV but calicivirus was not detected. The diagnosis of lymphocytic plasmacytic stomatitis was confirmed by the results of oral biopsies performed. Based upon the current literature, this patient was in stage III chronic terminal FIV disease.

To reduce the potential risk of severe side effects or death, the initial dose (14.8 mg/kg) of treatment selected was well below the calculated (120 mg/kg) optimal dose. Routine blood chemistry analyses were performed to observe indications of adverse reactions or side effects. Therapy consisted of intravenous injections of the drug, 3 times weekly, at approximately 14.8 mg/kg initially for 10 injections, increased to 29.67-37.1 mg/kg for the next 6 injections and then to doses varying from 75 mg/kg to 178 mg/kg for the remaining duration of therapy. A total of 29 injections (8,210 mg of drug) over a period of 100 days were given.

After the third dose of pMC540 injection, the tremendously strong mouth odor completely disappeared. A rapid dramatic improvement in oral stomatitis was observable by the 5th injection and bleeding virtually stopped by the 10th injection (Fig. 4.2a-b). At the end of the therapy, weight of the animal increased to 9.2 pounds and the owners noted a significantly enhanced activity and playfulness which was absent for the previous 6-8 months. The animal was able to eat well and the texture of its coat was significantly improved. There was a gradual increase in the time for the Cite® FeLV and FIV test to convert to positive and a decrease in the intensity of the positive color development was observed throughout the duration of treatment suggesting a reduction in viremia. However, these tests always remained positive. A gradual increase in the white blood cell count was also observed. This increased white blood cell count could be attributed to the pMC540-induced stimulation of the immune system or prevention of virus induced cell lysis. However, other possibilities such as vascular irritation or inflammation remain to be ruled out.

These results were obtained in somewhat less than ideal conditions because there were periodic gaps in the treatment due to unkept appointments, lack of sufficient quantities of available pMC540 and difficulties with venipuncture. Intravenous injections of this experimental drug caused a transient thickening of the vascular wall at the site of injections. However, the majority of the veins improved within a few weeks although the vessels appeared to retain some of the thickening for a month or more. It should also be mentioned, however, that biodistribution and clearance studies of pMC540 show that approximately 70% of this compound is cleared from the system within the first 6 hours.

Therefore, it is reasonable to predict that the observed beneficial response in these animals could have been significantly improved by changing the schedule of drug injections from three injections per week to perhaps single injection per day or every 6 to 8 hours. In other words, optimization of injection schedule is required for maximum therapeutic response. Alternatively, the formulation of the drug could be changed such that it is released more slowly over a period of time. Thus, a near complete eradication of viremia may be within the realm of possibilities requiring prolonged intensive therapy.

Except for the nausea and vomiting induced only by intraperitoneal injections and thickening of veins by intravenous injections, pMC540 was very easily tolerated up to a dose of 178 mg/kg as judged by the general well being of the treated animal and results

Fig. 4.2a.

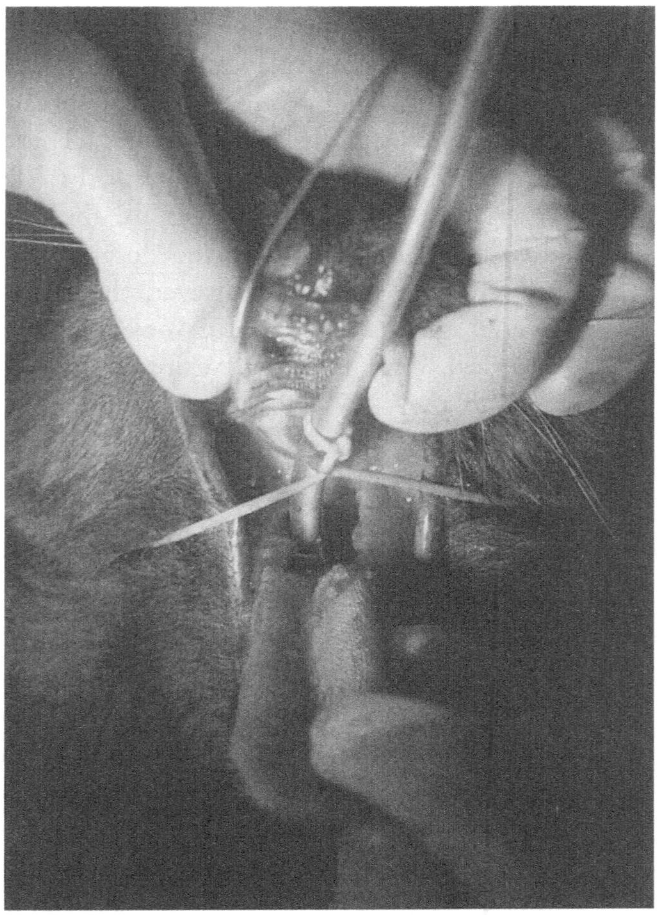

Fig. 4.2. Oral cavity of cat (a) immediately prior to the treatment and (b) approximately 10 days following onset of intravenous injections of preactivated merocyanine 540 (b, on opposite page). Reprinted with permission from J Vet Dent 1993; 10:9-13.

of the blood chemistry analysis during the course of treatment (Table 4.4). Virtually identical results were obtained when another cat suffering from generalized stomatitis, cervical line lesions, periodontal disease and spontaneous gingival bleeding with noticeable mouth odor was treated with pMC540.[5]

Thus, even though the data presented was obtained under less then ideal conditions, it clearly demonstrates the potential usefulness of the systemic use of pMC540 in the treatment of viral infection without producing serious side effects.

TREATMENT OF SIMIAN IMMUNE DEFICIENCY VIRUS INFECTION IN RHESUS MONKEY MODEL

As stated earlier in chapter 2, all HIV and SIV related experiments were carried out in collaboration with Dr. Tran Chan, Department of Virology and Immunology and Center for AIDS Research, Southwest Foundation for Biomedical Research, San Antonio, Texas. Experiments were designed to assess the effects of pMC540 in a rhesus monkey model for AIDS. For this purpose, a rhesus macaque weighing approximately 10 kilograms was

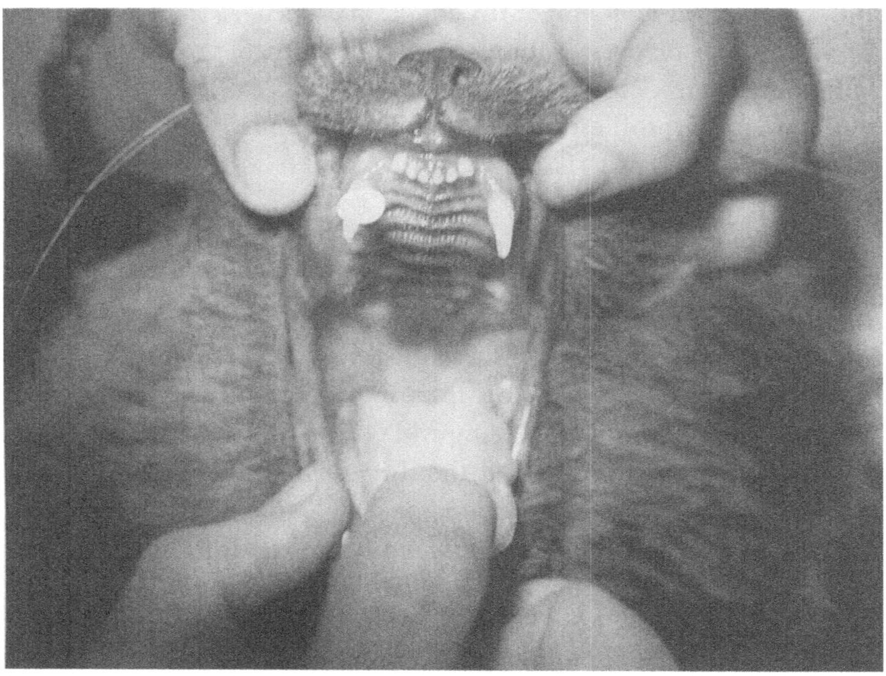

Fig. 4.2b.

Table 4.4. Laboratory results case no. 1 (Basic results are provided, more extensive profiles were evaluated)

DATE	RBC	HCT	WBC	HGB	BUN	SGOT	SGPT	GLU	CREA	FeLV	FIV
2/25	5.31	27.7	5.4	10.5	10.6	20	34	137	1.6	+	+
3/2	6.59	30.6	5.5	10.9	11.2	20	10	147	1.3	+	+
3/11	7.90	45.8	7.8	12.8	13	20	10	139	1.1	+	+
3/18	9.38	43.9	6.2	11.6	14	20	10	114	1.4	+	+
3/26	8.30	36.9	8.8	11.9	13.1	20	17	111	1.1	+	+
4/8	9.27	34.9	9.2	11.6	9.7	20	11	123	1.3	+	+
4/17	8.18	32.1	10.8	8.9	10.8	20	10	121	1.3	+	+
5/15	8.30	31.4	6.9	8.9	12.1	20	33	141	1.7	+	+
6/1	4.71	27	8.5	8.6	11.8	21	23	131	1.4	+	+
6/5	4.73	23.9	8.6	8.3	15.7	21	12	105	1.5	+	+

Note: A gradual increase in the time for the Cite® FeLV and FIV test to convert to positive was seen throughout the treatment, but at no time did the tests become negative. Reprinted with permission from J Vet Dent 1993; 10:9-13.

quarantined for 40 days and then a blood sample was obtained to establish the baseline values of the markers listed below: lymphocyte surface markers using anti-Leu-3a, anti-Leu-2a, anti-Leu-5, anti-Leu-4, anti-Leu-M3, anti-Leu-11, anti-Leu-19 and anti-Leu-12 antibodies; helper / suppressor ratio; in vitro proliferation response to PHA, Con-A and PWM; natural killer cell activity; CBC and SMAC-28 profiles; and plasma, serum and PBMC were also frozen for future use. This monkey was then inoculated with an infectious dose of $SIV_{(mac\ 251)}$.

The establishment of SIV-infection was confirmed by virus isolation. The rhesus monkey was then treated with pMC540 (28 intravenous injections; cumulative dose of 580mg/kg) over a period of 60 days. The monkey was bled every 2 weeks for serological assays such as immunoblot, immunofluorescence, p24 antigen-capture assay, viral isolation using MT-4 cells and PCR to pinpoint the time of seroconversion and the time of in-vitro virus isolation.

After 28 intravenous injections of pMC540, the treatment was terminated because the virus could no longer be isolated from the monkey's blood. Toxicity data suggest that pMC540 was well tolerated as determined by CBC and SMAC-28 profiles and the general well being of the animal. In particular, the values of lactate dehydrogenase and creatinine phosphokinase enzymes, indicative of insult to the heart muscle, did not show a significant change. Nine months after the termination of the treatment the virus still could not be isolated from the blood and the monkey did not show any AIDS-like symptoms. In an attempt to identify the target organ of toxicity another rhesus monkey (which was morbid and destined to be euthanized) was infused with escalating doses of pMC540. No discernible toxicity was observed up to a dose of 120 mg/kg. However, when the dose was increased to 160 mg/kg, the monkey died 3 days later. The cause of death, determined by the attending pathologist, was due to tubular necrosis. It was recognized that clear interpretation of these results may have been compromised due to the advanced disease state, concomitant parasitic infections and the cumulative drug dose effect. However, the general well being of the animal during treatment and the absence of gross abnormalities in the autopsy report lends support for further detailed investigation of the toxicological effects of pMC540.

It is recognized however, that AIDS is a complex disease and even though we have acquired extensive knowledge of the molecular characteristics of the human immunodeficiency virus, a great deal of knowledge regarding the pathophysiological basis of the profound and irreversible immune depression that follows this retrolentiviral infection remains obscure. Thus, in view of the in vivo anti-viral effects of pMC540, significant questions such as, how this agent controls the HIV replication, what are the correlates of protection, can pMC540 target HIV in reservoirs like lymph nodes, effect of pMC540 on reconstitution of the immune system etc., remain to be answered. Even so, most important of all these is the question, can pMC540 (or any other agent) truly control or terminate HIV replication and simultaneously destroy the HIV infected cells i.e. the virus producing factory? If the answer to this question is 'no' then asking all other questions may only help to add to the existing knowledge base with little or no immediate benefit to the patients who are dying everyday. But what about pMC540? Is it effective in the inactivation of HIV as well as in destroying the virus producing factory, the infected cell? The answer to this question is that all experimental data point to the fact that this agent appears to be capable of destroying the HIV as well as HIV-infected cells without producing serious side effects. Thus, this very promising antiviral candidate is worthy of further investigation.

PRECLINICAL ACTIVITY OF pMC540 AGAINST BREAST CANCER

In this section, the activity of pMC540 and one of its chemically synthesized isolate merodantoin against human breast tumor xenografts will be discussed. However, before proceeding with this discussion it is important to briefly review the presently available treatments for breast cancer.

CURRENT TREATMENTS OF HUMAN BREAST CANCER

Breast cancer is unique in being sensitive to a wide variety of chemotherapeutic and hormonal agents. Thus, the current treatments for breast cancer involve the use of many endocrine manipulations, or the use of antitumor agents principally the alkylating agents Cytoxan, thio-TEPA, mitomycin C, and L-PAM; the topoisomerase II/intercalators, doxorubicin and mitoxantrone; the antimetabolites 5-fluorouracil and methotrexate; and the vinca alkaloids vincristine and vinblastine.

However, these agents by themselves or in combination have not produced entirely satisfactory results. To maximize the intensity with which these agents can be employed, they have been used with hematopoietic growth factors or autotransplantation or with different schedules of administration. Even so, most investigators have limited expectations for these standard chemotherapeutic drugs. They believe that entirely new active agents are needed. Thus, a vigorous drug discovery program has produced new clinically promising agents such as Taxol and Taxotere, which act as tubulin superstabilizer, and Navelbine which acts as a tubulin destabilizer; Anthrapyrazoles CI 941, a DNA intercalator; Edaterxate, an antifolate compound, and Topotecan and CPT-11 which mediate their effect via inhibition of topoisomerase I.

The objective response rates for Taxol and doxorubicin have been 40% to 50% in good risk stage IV patients.[6,7] Although it is not too unrealistic to aim for very high levels of partial and complete responses, the need for new agents for breast cancer treatment is widely recognized. Is it even possible that any single chemical agent will ever be an effective treatment for cancer? The answer is clearly 'yes' which is evident by the fact that at present, vigorous efforts drug discovery programs of the National Cancer Institute and pharmaceutical industry are fertile, and chemotherapy armamentarium for breast cancer is expected to double providing more than 30 active cytotoxic agents each with high expectations.

In finding a new therapeutic agent one of the requirements is that the new agent has to be better than those already available. Therefore, it is important to ask once again what are the most desirable properties one must strive for in a new chemotherapeutic agent? The ideal goal of cancer therapy requires that treatment must be effective in destroying the cancer and treatment must spare the host. The sparing of the host is the most important point as discussed in the beginning of this chapter. Our experience (at this stage) with unique compounds such as preactivated merocyanine 540 (pMC540) and merodantoin provides evidence that indeed it is entirely possible to develop new chemotherapeutic agents that are effective against different types of cancer yet they spare the host. In so doing, progress towards achieving the ideal goal of cancer therapy has been moved forward.

HUMAN TUMOR XENOGRAFTS IN NUDE MICE

As stated earlier, the main goal of any cancer chemotherapy is elimination of tumor and preservation of normal cells and tissues. While in vitro data is essential for initial screening of a new chemotherapeutic agent, its true efficacy can only be determined in target host. The physiological and clinical significance of in vitro observations are often controversial and difficult to interpret due to lack of host-related determinants that affect tumor behavior in vivo. Since human experimentation with experimental drugs can only occur after substantial in vitro and in vivo data regarding the efficacy and toxicity of a given compound has been accumulated, animal models are used to mimic in vivo conditions of the host. The human tumor xenografts in nude mice are regarded as one of the best models available for the study of human tumor biology. The experiments can be performed under reproducible and controlled conditions. Xenografts provide a unique and renewable source of tumor material for biological studies, and this model is presently considered to be a powerful tool in the development of new cancer therapies. This view is strengthened by the fact that there is a positive correlation between drug responses in the xenografts and those in the original patient's tumors. In a study involving all cases reported in literature, it was reported that in the majority of comparisons (125 out of 138), the response in xenografts and that in patients appeared to correlate well.[8] However, it is important to note that in animal models relevant characteristics such as growth rate, cell cycle parameters, metastatic potential, invasive properties, origin of stroma, pharmacokinetics and metabolism in tumor-bearing host are likely to be different from the cancer patient and a direct translation of results to humans is not possible in each and every case.

For the studies of the effect of pMC540 and merodantoin against human breast cancer, an athymic mouse model was chosen since this model is most commonly used for breast cancer research. This model has existed since early 1960 and remains the most popular heterotransplantation host.[9] More recently, the SCID mouse has offered a new model for heterotransplantation. Comparative studies of nude mice and SCID mice have shown a generally higher take rate in SCID mice for certain tumor types. In our hands, however, the take rate of breast tumors has been virtually 100%, justifying the use of athymic (nude) mice.

Effect of pMC540 and Merodantoin on MCF-7 Human Breast Cancer Xenografts

As described in chapter 2, three photoproducts, merocil, meroxazole and merodantoin were isolated from pMC540 and characterized. Meroxazole turned out to be a nontoxic component as determined by in vitro cytotoxicity assays described in chapter 5. However, merocil and merodantoin were quite potent and represent approximately 99% of the cytotoxicity observed with pMC540. Merodantoin was easily synthesized in 50 gram quantities in our laboratories and used for subsequent in vitro and in vivo studies. In vitro experiments revealed that both pMC540 and merodantoin were quite effective in killing the human breast adenocarcinoma MCF-7 cells. These in vitro studies were performed to assess the dose effect of pMC540 and merodantoin on human breast cancer cells. Both pMC540 and merodantoin produced a dose dependent cytotoxicity in human breast cancer MCF-7 cells (Figs. 4.3 and 4.4).

Cytotoxicity induced by merodantoin was more rapid as compared to the gradual increase in cytotoxicity observed with pMC540. Next, effect of these compounds on the inhibition of clonogenic growth was determined. Results show (Table 4.5) that clonogenic growth of MCF-7 cells was aborted by the presence of pMC540 (40 μg/ml or 70.2 μM for 48 hr) and merodantoin (10 μg/ml or 41.3 μM for 48 hr). Therefore, after establishing the in vitro effectiveness, the in vivo activity of merodantoin and pMC540 was evaluated against MCF-7 human breast tumors transplanted into athymic mice.

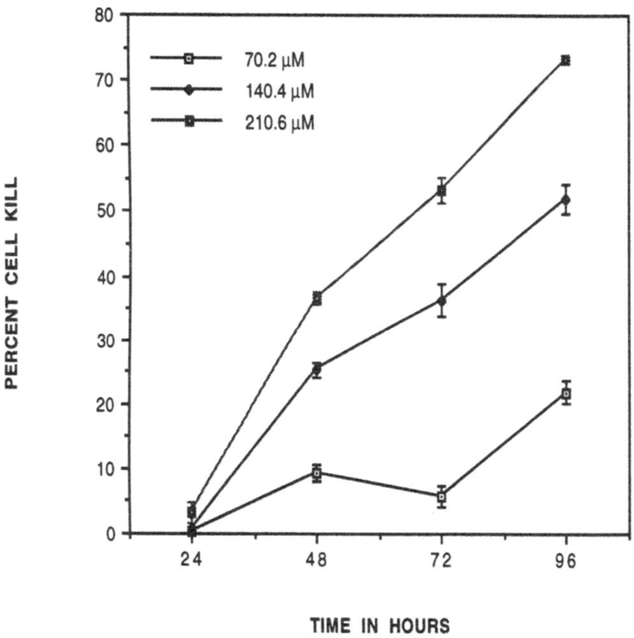

Fig. 4.3. Dose-effect curves of pMC540 against MCF-7 cells. Cells (5 x 10 ^{4} cells/ml) were treated with indicated doses of pMC540 (1.0 μg/ml = 1.755 μM). After incubation at 37° C for 24, 48, 72 or 96 hours, the cell viability was determined by MTT assay. Results (mean ± standard error of the mean) of three separate experiments performed in quadruplicate are shown. Reprinted with permission from Cancer 1994; 74:1725-1732.

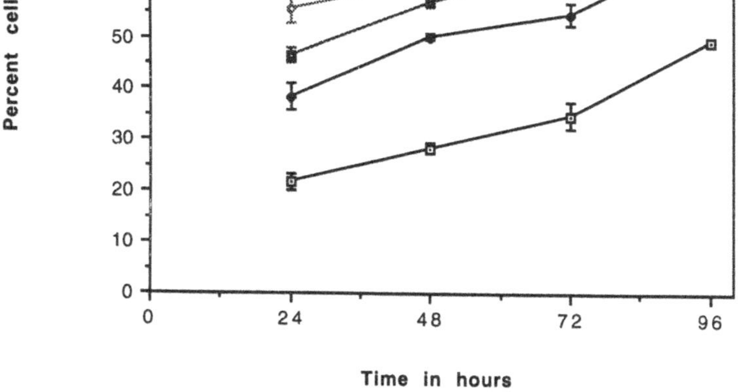

Fig. 4.4. Dose-effect curves of merodantoin against MCF-7 cells. Cells (5 x 10^4 cells/ml) were treated with indicated doses of merodantoin (1.0 μg/ml = 4.13 μM). After incubation at 37° C for 24, 48, 72 or 96 hours, the cell viability was determined by MTT assay. Results (mean ± standard error of the mean) of three separate experiments performed in quadruplicate are shown. Reprinted with permission from Cancer 1994; 74: 1725-1732.

Establishment of Solid MCF-7 Breast Tumors in Nude Mice

To assess the effect of pMC540 and merodantoin against solid breast tumors, human breast adenocarcinoma MCF-7 cells were grown as solid tumors in athymic nude mice with exogenously supplied estradiol support. Briefly, 3 days prior to the injection of MCF-7 cells into nude mice, 17b-estradiol, in 60-day release pellet form, was transplanted subcutaneously. On the fourth day 1 x 10^7 MCF-7 cells were injected subcutaneously. Solid tumors appeared within 45 days. Resulting solid tumors were excised, cut into small pieces (2x2 mm) and transplanted into native athymic mice in which slow release estradiol pellets had been transplanted. A group of separately maintained nude mice served as a source of solid breast tumors for all subsequent experiments.

Effect of Intratumoral Injection of pMC540

Transplanted tumors (5x5 mm) were allowed to grow. When the tumor size increased to 7x6 mm, 8 intratumoral injections of pMC540 (250 mg/kg) were given over a period of 16 days. After 6 doses of treatment the tumor necrosis in the central part of the tumor was clearly visible. Continued treatment caused a significant ($p < 0.001$) regression of all treated tumors (Table 4.6) and tumors could not be detected in 3 of the mice at the end of treatment. Untreated tumors continued to grow and reached an average area of 10.5 cm^2 at the end of 16 days. This treatment was easily tolerated without any

Table 4.5. Effect of pMC540 and merodantoin on clonogenic growth of MCF-7 breast cancer cells

Clonogenic Growth in MCF-7 Cells Treatment	No. of Colonies
Untreated	204
*pMC540 (140.4 µM for 24 hours)	87
pMC540 (70.2 µM for 48 hours)	0
pMC540 (140.4 µM for 48 hours)	0
MD (41.3 µM for 24 hours)	3
MD (41.3 µM for 48 hours)	0
MD (61.95 µM for 48 hours)	0

MCF-7 cells (5 x 10^5 cells/ml) were treated with pMC540 (70.2 µM and 140.4 µM) or MD (20.6 µM, 41.3 µM, and 61.95 µM) for 24 to 48 hours. After the incubation period, cells were plated in clonogenic growth medium. To prevent the attachment of cells to the plate, a layer of 3% methylcellulose was placed in the bottom of the wells. Colonies consisting of 50 or more cells were counted on day 7. Latent growth was monitored for 15 days. Results of a representative experiment carried out in triplicate are shown. *pMC540 = preactivated merocyanine 540; MD = merodantoin. Reprinted with permission from Cancer 1994; 74:1725-1732.

observable signs of discomfort or toxicity. The weight of treated and control animals did not vary significantly. In fact, the average weight of the treated group was slightly higher then the controls, probably due to low tumor burden. These data demonstrate the susceptibility of solid human breast tumor xenografts to the cytotoxic action of photoproducts in pMC540. Next, the effect of systemically injected pMC540 and merodantoin on solid human breast tumor xenografts was examined.

SYSTEMIC TREATMENT OF BREAST TUMOR XENOGRAFTS

Intramuscular injections of pMC540 (250 mg/kg) or merodantoin (75 mg/kg) were given in the hind limbs on alternate days for a period of 40 days. The control group of animals received vehicle (dimethyl sulfoxide) only. Results of this study demonstrate (Fig. 4.5) that a brief period of treatment with merodantoin caused 98% inhibition of tumor growth (Table 4.7) whereas treatment with pMC540 caused a 43% inhibition of tumor growth as compared to the untreated controls (Table 4.8).

In the merodantoin treated group 50% of the animals did not present a palpable tumor at the end of the treatment. Tumor growth curves for MCF-7 xenografts show that merodantoin appears to cause a rapid tumor regression in these small tumors mimicking early stages of tumor growth. These studies clearly show that both pMC540 and merodantoin were effective in controlling the growth of solid human breast tumor xenografts.

Table 4.6. Effect of intratumor injections of pMC540 on MCF-7 breast tumor transplanted into athymic mice

Treatment Group	Dose	Tumor Area, cm^2 (on last day)	Tumor Weight, g (mean±SD)	Tumor Volume, cm^3 (mean±SD)	% TGI
Control (n=7)	–	10.460±5.244	0.719±0.4326	0.4981±0.4399	
pMC540 (n=7)*	250 mg/kg	2.120±2.040	0.2645±0.1116	0.068±0.077	63.21
		P = .0026	*P* = .0056	*P* = .00256	

Route of drug administration: intratumor, 8 doses on alternate days. Size of tumor implanted: 5 x 5 mm; treatment initiated when tumor size was 7 x 6 mm. *Three animals did not show any palpable tumors at the end of the treatment. %TGI indicates percent tumor growth inhibition, calculated by using the formula %TGI = $100(1-W_t/W_c)$, where W_t and W_c are the mean weights of the treated and control tumors, respectively. Reprinted with permission from Cancer 1994; 74:1725-1732.

Fig. 4.5.

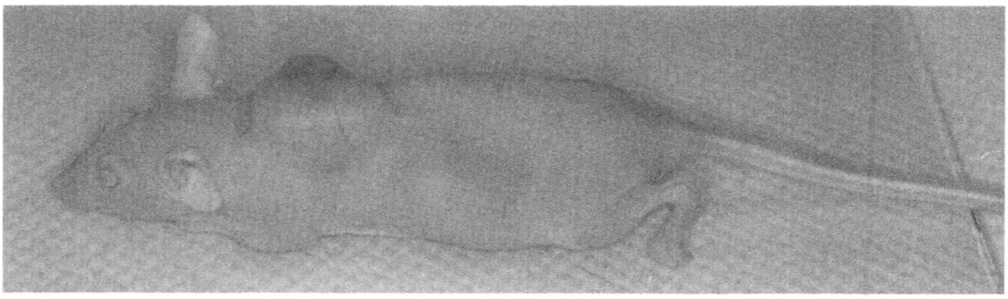

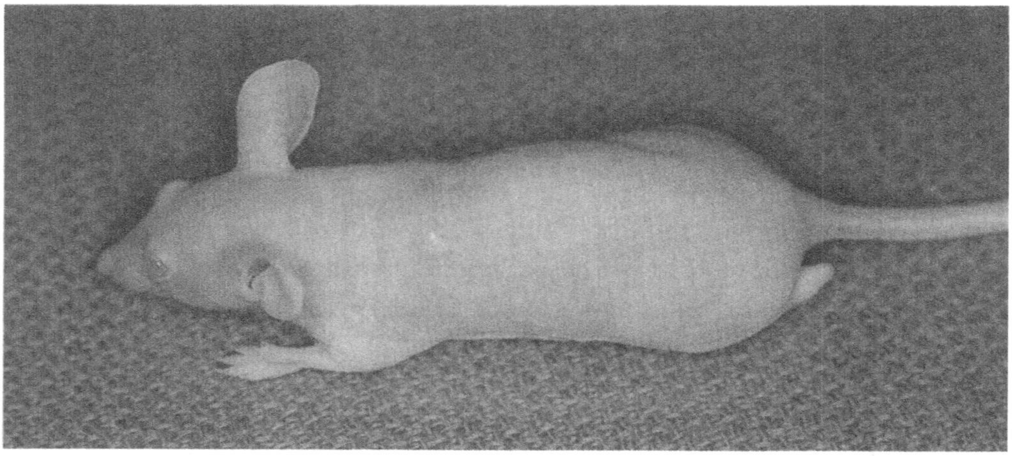

Fig. 4.5. Photographs of athymic mice bearing human breast tumor. Top: control, treated with vehicle only; bottom: treated with merodantoin (75 kg/mg) on alternate days for 40 days. Reprinted with permission from Cancer 1994; 74:1725-1732.

Table 4.7. Effect of merodantoin on the growth of MCF-7 tumor

Treatment Group	Dose	Tumor Area (cm^2)	Tumor Weight (g)	Tumor Volume (cm^3)	%TGI
Control* (n = 10)	Vehicle only	10.780 ± 1.44	0.797 ± 0.141	0.800 ± 0.141	
Merodantoin (n = 6)	75 mg/kg	0.211 ± 0.104 (*P* = .0001)	0.011 ± 0.004 (*P* = .0009)	ND	98.62

*Implantation size, approximately 2x2 mm. Treatments with merodantoin were given on alternate days via intramuscular injections for 40 days. Final tumor size measurements were made on day 40. %TGI was calculated as described in legend for Table 4.6. Reprinted with permission from Cancer 1994; 74:1725-1732.

Treatment of Breast Tumor Xenografts with Combination of Tamoxifen and pMC540

Human adenocarcinoma MCF-7 cells used in this study were positive for estrogen receptors with estrogen receptor site binding concentration in the range of 236 fmol/mg protein.[10] Tamoxifen has been successfully used in the treatment of estrogen positive breast cancer and it is the antihormonal agent of choice.[11,12] In a previous in vitro study, we reported that a combination of preactivated photofrin II and tamoxifen produced enhanced killing of breast cancer cells in a synergistic manner.[10] Encouraged by these findings, we elected to expand our studies to include the determination of the effects of tamoxifen plus pMC540 or merodantoin. Results from these studies show (Table 4.8) that a combination of tamoxifen plus pMC540 increased the tumor growth inhibition from 43% to 67%. However, at the concentration used, tamoxifen alone failed to inhibit the growth of breast tumor xenografts. This lack of tumor growth inhibition probably occurred because the serum level ratio of estrogen and anti-estrogen was not complementary. It is well established that the growth rate of MCF-7 xenografts is estradiol concentration dependent.[13,14]

Table 4.8. Effect of pMC540, tamoxifen and tamoxifen + pMC540 on the growth of MCF-7 tumor

Treatment Group	Dose	Tumor Area (cm^2)	Tumor Weight (g)	Tumor Volume (cm^3)	%TGI
Control* (n = 10)	Vehicle only	10.780 ± 1.44	0.797 ± 0.141	0.800 ± 0.141	
pMC540 (n = 10)	250 mg/kg	5.030 ± 1.02 (*P* = .0044)**	0.455 ± 0.123 (*P* = .0882)	0.471 ± 0.118 (*P* = .0903)	42.91
Tamoxifen (n = 10)	5-mg pellet/ mouse	11.090 ± 1.700 (*P* = .8909)	1.059 ± 0.177 (*P* = .2604)	1.058 ± 0.172 (*P* = .2609)	
Tamoxifen plus pMC540 (n = 10)	5-mg pellet + 100 mg/kg	3.310 ± 0.710 (*P* = .0002)	0.263 ± 0.071 (*P* = .029)	0.311 ± 0.077 (*P* = .0069)	67.0

*Implantation size approximately 2x2 mm. Treatments with pMC540 were given on alternate days via intramuscular injections for 40 days. Final tumor size assessments were made on day 40. %TGI was calculated as described in legend for Table 4.6. Reprinted with permission from Cancer 1994; 74:1725-1732.

The dose of estradiol (1.7 mg pellets) used in this study is known to produce serum levels of 900 pg/ml and tamoxifen (5 mg pellets) is known to produce very low (4-5 ng/ml) serum levels.[15] For effective tumor growth inhibition, doses of estradiol (0.5-1.0 mg) producing serum levels of 300-600 pg/ml and tamoxifen producing serum levels of 40-50 ng/ml have been used.[16] Thus, the observed lack of tumor growth inhibition by tamoxifen alone is explained by noncomplementary serum levels of estrogen and anti-estrogen. Nonetheless it is clear from the data presented that systemically injected pMC540 and merodantoin were effective in controlling the growth of solid human breast tumor xenografts mimicking early stages of tumor growth.

Treatment of Established Breast Tumor Xenografts with pMC540 and Merodantoin

To further build upon the data described thus far, the effect of pMC540 and merodantoin was determined against established human breast tumor xenografts mimicking the late stages of breast tumor growth. For these experiments, solid MCF-7 breast tumors were transplanted into nude mice as described above and then allowed to grow for a period of 10-12 days. Intramuscular injections of pMC540 and merodantoin were then given on alternate days for a period of 40 days. Tumor sizes were measured weekly. Growth curves of tumors treated with pMC540 (250 mg/kg) show (Fig. 4.6) that this treatment prevented further growth of established tumors whereas untreated tumors continued to grow. Addition of tamoxifen to this treatment regimen did not produce appreciable enhancement of tumor growth inhibition. At the end of the 40 day treatment, overall tumor growth inhibition amounted to 84% in pMC540 treated group and 93% in pMC540 plus tamoxifen group (Table 4.9). Similar results (Fig. 4.7 and Table 4.10) were obtained in a group treated with merodantoin as well as merodantoin plus tamoxifen. These results suggest that both merodantoin and pMC540 were also effective in controlling the growth of established breast tumor xenografts.

TREATMENT OF ESTABLISHED BREAST TUMOR XENOGRAFTS UNDER THE CONDITIONS OF ESTROGEN DEPRIVATION

To determine the effect of pMC540 and merodantoin against established tumors under the conditions of estrogen deprivation,

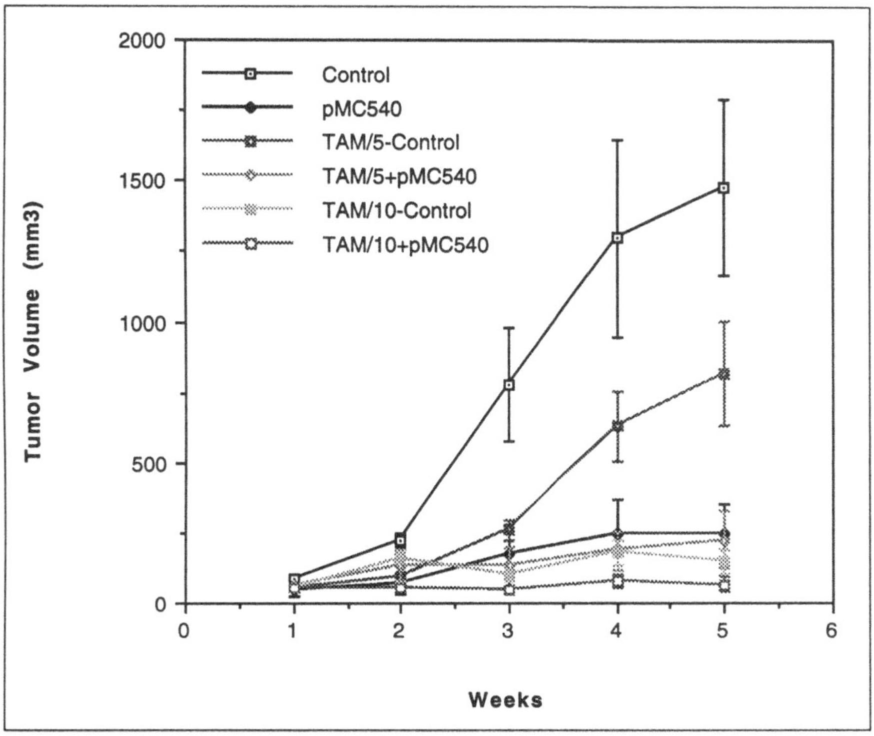

Fig. 4.6. Growth curves (mean ± S.E.M.) of established MCF-7 tumor xenografts in the continuous presence of estrogen (control) and treated with pMC540 (250 mg/kg), tamoxifen (TAM) 5mg and 10 mg pellets, and TAM plus pMC540. Alternate-day treatment of mice was initiated 10-12 days after tumor implantation. There were 10 mice per group. Reprinted with permission from In Vivo 1995; 9:103-108.

Table 4.9. Effect of pMC540 and tamoxifen on established breast tumors

Treatment	Dose	Area (mm²)	Weight	Vol. (mm³)	% TGI
Control	Vehicle only	162.5 ± 22.9	1.283 ± 0.119	1475.8 ±314.21	
pMC540	250 mg/kg	51.7 ± 7.0	0.326 ± 0.062	240.3 ± 40.8	74.6
TAM	5 mg	92.1 ± 13.1	1.059 ± 0.177	821.2 ± 184.8	18.5
TAM	10 mg	33.0 ± 8.0	0.200 ± 0.045	150.2 ± 44.3	84.6
TAM + pMC540	5 mg + 250 mg/kg	43.1 ± 14.1	0.227 ± 0.118	226.8 ± 100.1	82.5
TAM + pMC540	10 mg + 250 mg/kg	18.7 ± 6.2	0.088 ± 0.031	67.4 ± 26.8	93.2

Implantation tumor size approximately 2 x 2 mm. Tumors were allowed to grow to an approximate size of 5 x 6 mm (approximately 8-10 days). Treatment with pMC540 was given on alternate days via intramuscular injection for 30 days. Final tumor size assessment was made on day 34. % TGI indicates percent tumor growth inhibition, calculated using the formula $\%TGI = 100\,(1 - W_t/W_c)$, where W_t and W_c are the mean weights of the treated and controlled tumors respectively. Reprinted with permission from In Vivo 1995; 9:103-108.

MCF-7 breast tumors were allowed to grow for 10-12 days in the presence of exogenous estradiol. However, prior to the initiation of drug treatment, the estrogen pellets were surgically removed. Then, intramuscular injections of pMC540 (250 mg/kg) or merodantoin (75 mg/kg) in the presence or absence of tamoxifen were given in the hind limbs on alternate days for 40 days. Under

Table 4.10. Effect of merodantoin and tamoxifen on established breast tumors

Treatment	Dose	Area (mm^2)	Weight (gm)	Vol. (mm^3)	% TGI
Control	Vehicle only	162.5 ± 22.9	1.283 ± 0.119	1475.8 ±314.21	
MD	75 mg/kg	31.9 ± 5.2	0.191 ± 0.048	119.1 ± 29.8	84.6
TAM	5 mg pellet	92.1 ± 13.1	1.059 ± 0.177	821.2 ± 184.8	18.5
TAM	10 mg pellet	33.0 ± 8.0	0.200 ± 0.045	150.2 ± 44.3	84.6
TAM + MD	5 mg + 75 mg/kg	25.3 ± 8.6	0.136 ± 0.047	115.8 ± 43.7	89
TAM + MD	10 mg + 75 mg/kg	18.2 ± 6.8	0.086 ± 0.033	64.98 ± 3.41	93.1

Implantation tumor size approximately 2 x 2 mm. Tumors were allowed to grow to an approximate size of 5 x 6 mm (approximately 8-10 days). Treatment with pMC540 was given on alternate days via intramuscular injection for 30 days. Final tumor size assessment was made on day 34. %TGI was calculated as described in legend for table 4.9. Reprinted with permission from In Vivo 1995; 9:103-108.

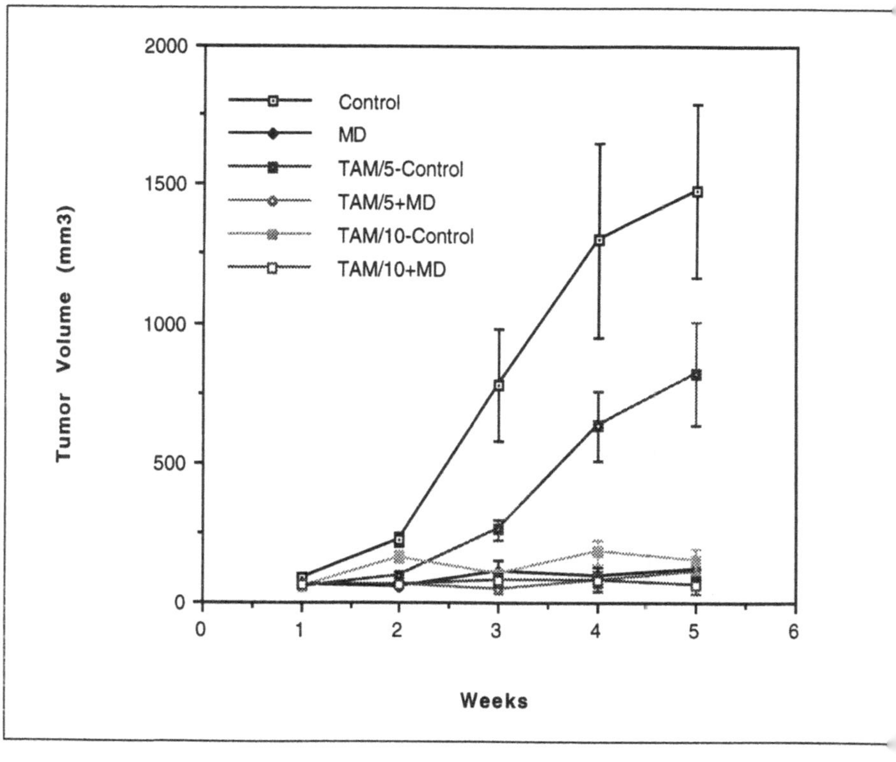

Fig. 4.7. Growth curves (mean ± S.E.M.) of established MCF-7 tumor xenografts in the continuous presence of estrogen (control) and treated with merodantoin (MD; 75 mg/kg), tamoxifen (TAM) 5 mg and 10 mg pellets, and TAM plus merodantoin (MD). Alternate-day treatment of mice was initiated 10-12 days after tumor implantation. There were 10 mice per group. Reprinted with permission from In Vivo 1995; 9:103-108.

the estrogen withdrawal conditions all tumors began to regress spontaneously and treatment with pMC540 or merodantoin did not produce a dramatic difference in the rate of tumor regression (Figs. 4.8 and 4.9). It is noteworthy here that the growth of MCF-7 tumors is known to be estrogen dependent. During the course of these experiments unexpected results were observed; a combined treatment with tamoxifen (10 mg, 60 day pellets) and pMC540 or merodantoin caused stimulation of tumor growth. This effect was less pronounced in the case of merodantoin and occurred only under the conditions of estrogen deprivation. The mechanism of this stimulatory effect is unclear but appears to resemble the transient growth stimulatory activity of tamoxifen. This process probably involves initial binding to estrogen receptors followed by its translocation to the nucleus, resulting in an induction of a brief burst of estrogenic activity prior to the onset of anti-estrogenic effect.[17] A similar mechanism operating in breast cancer patients

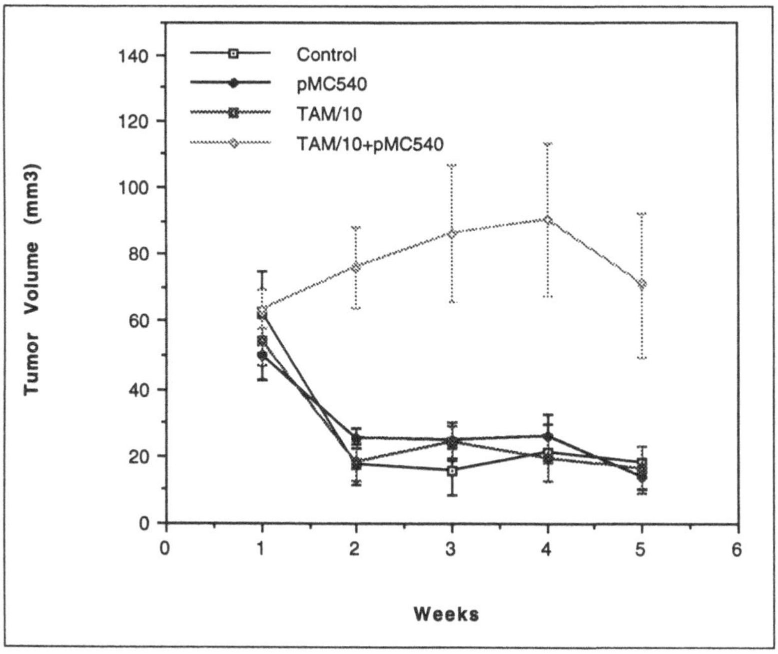

Fig. 4.8. Growth curves (mean ±S.E.M.) of established MCF-7 tumor xenografts under the estradiol deprived conditions (control) and treated with pMC540 (250 mg/kg), tamoxifen (TAM) 5 mg and 10 mg pellets, and TAM plus pMC540. Alternate-day treatment of mice was initiated 10-12 days after tumor implantation. There were 10 mice per group. Reprinted with permission from In Vivo 1995; 9:103-108.

where disease "flairs" upon initiation of tamoxifen therapy has been reported.[18] Nonetheless, the treatment of estrogen dependent breast tumors in the absence of exogenous estrogen with pMC540 and merodantoin was not successful in causing a complete eradication of these tumors even though they were regressing due to lack of exogenously supplied estrogen. In view of these observations it was important to determine whether treatment of estrogen receptor negative breast tumors with these agents would produce the dramatic response seen in the treatment of estrogen receptor positive tumors. Thus, the following experiments were carried out.

Treatment of Estrogen Receptor Negative Established Human Breast Tumor Xenografts

To determine whether pMC540 and merodantoin would be effective in controlling the growth of estrogen receptor negative breast tumors, a human breast cancer cell line MDA-MB-435 was

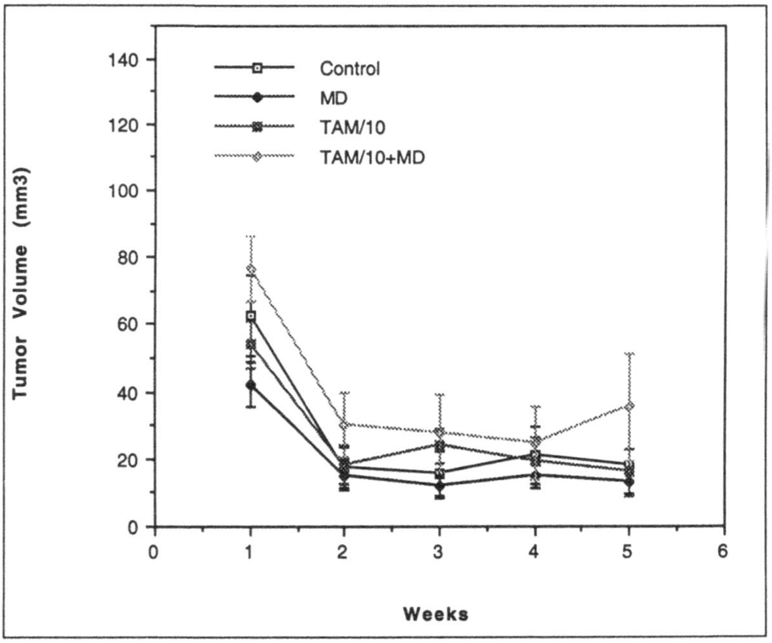

Fig. 4.9. Growth curves (mean ±S.E.M.) of established MCF-7 tumor xenografts under the estradiol deprived conditions (control) and treated with merodantoin (MD; 75 mg/kg), tamoxifen (TAM) 5 mg and 10 mg pellets, and TAM plus merodantoin (MD). Alternate-day treatment of mice was initiated 10-12 days after tumor implantation. There were 10 mice per group. Reprinted with permission from In Vivo 1995; 9:103-108.

used. These cells were transplanted into athymic mice without the support of exogenous estradiol. Resulting solid tumors were serially transplanted into native athymic mice and then allowed to grow from an approximate size of 2 x 2 mm to 5 x 5 mm. Athymic mice (n = 6) bearing established MDA-MB-435 breast tumors were treated with pMC540 (250 mg/kg) or merodantoin (75 mg/kg). Intramuscular injections were given on alternate days for a period of 40 days. Data from these experiments show that both agents caused a 59% inhibition of tumor growth as compared to the untreated controls in which tumors continued to grow (Fig. 4.10). Treatment with merodantoin caused an initial tumor regression amounting to approximately 34% reduction in tumor volume. However, the observed tumor regression did not continue. After the first two weeks of treatment tumor growth adopted a stationary phase. These data suggest that although pMC540 and merodantoin were effective in controlling the growth of estrogen dependent breast tumors, the extent of overall growth inhibition was significantly reduced in the estrogen receptor negative tumors suggesting that either the estrogen receptor negative breast tumors are less responsive to these agents or a different drug dose regimen

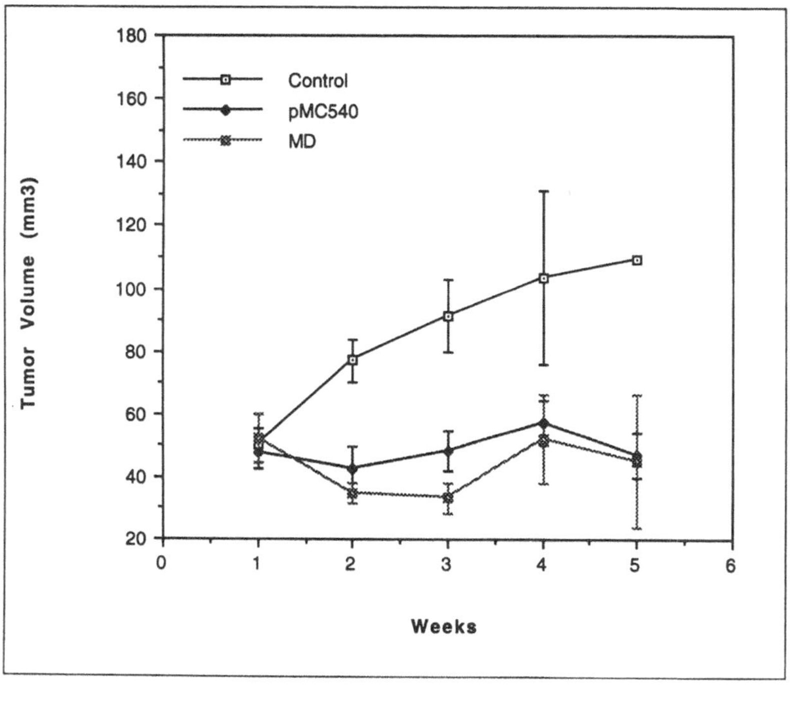

Fig. 4.10. Growth curves (mean ± S.E.M.) of established MDA-MB-435 tumor xenografts under the conditions: control and treated with pMC540 (250 mg/kg) or merodantoin (MD; 75 mg/kg) are shown. Alternate day injections were given 10-12 days after tumor implantation. There were 10 mice per group. Reprinted with permission from In Vivo 1995; 9:103-108.

is required. Thus, drug dose and schedule of drug injections need to be optimized.

EFFECT OF pMC540 AND MERODANTOIN ON TUMOR INVASIVENESS

Tumor metastasis is the major cause of morbidity for breast cancer patients. It therefore follows that therapeutic treatment of metastasis is extraordinarily important for effective control of cancer. Cancer metastasis consists of multiple sequential steps that include: 1) release of tumor cells from primary site; 2) entrance into blood circulation (intravasation); 3) access to the target organ; 4) extravasation (penetration into parenchyma of the organ) and 5) growth in the secondary site.[19-22] In many cases, metastasis occurs from established metastases. Invasion is one of the most characteristic steps during the cascade of metastasis. Thus, prevention of invasion would be useful in the control of metastasis. Invasion consists of three steps: 1) adhesion to the extracellular matrix; 2) degradation of extracellular matrix by several kinds of hydrolases and 3) migration through the extracellular matrix.[23, 24] Many studies have demonstrated that the inhibition of any of these steps results in the prevention of metastases.[25-29]

In order to determine the effectiveness of pMC540 or merodantoin in inhibiting the tumor cell invasiveness, an in vitro model employing NIH/3T3 mouse fibroblast cells (noninvasive control) and invasive human fibrosarcoma HT-1080 cells was used. This in vitro invasion assay was performed in the membrane invasion culture system using a polycarbonate filter containing 8 μm pores coated with a reconstituted basement membrane matrix (Matrigel invasion chamber) available from Becton Dickson. Invasion chambers were first rehydrated for 2 hours at room temperature by adding 2 ml of warm Dulbecco's minimal essential medium (DMEM) serum-free growth medium. After the rehydration period, the serum-free medium was removed and replaced with 2 ml of DMEM containing 1.8×10^5 HT-1080 cells in 0.1% bovine serum albumin. The bottom of the wells was filled with 2.5 ml of DMEM supplemented with 10% fetal calf serum. Cells were allowed to attach for 2 hours at 37°C and then exposed to different concentrations of pMC540 or merodantoin added to the upper chamber containing cells. The control chambers received vehicle control only. After 4 hours of incubation (determined in a preliminary time response experiment) cells were removed from the wells and membrane surfaces were wiped thoroughly with cotton swabs. Filters were removed from chambers, placed on a slide with bottom side up and stained with diffQuick staining solution. Results form a typical preliminary experiment show (Fig 4.11) that a 4 hour treatment with 30 μg/ml (52.65 μM) of pMC540 caused a virtually complete inhibition of HT-1080 cell invasion. A similar treatment of cells with merodantoin (103.3 mM for 72 hours) resulted in a 47% inhibition of cell migration. The comparative reduction in migration obtained in the presence of merodantoin apprears to be due to the lack of uniform distribution of lipophilic merodantoin in water. This would be consistent withour observations that the performance of merodantoin is significantly superior under in vivo conditons.

The data presented clearly indicates that pMC540 and merodantoin were effective in causing a significant ($p < 0.001$) inhibition of tumor cell invasiveness in the in vitro model.

In vivo effects of pMC540 and merodantoin on tumor metastasis

It has been reported that estrogen receptor negative human breast cancer MDA-MB-435 cells spontaneously metastasize from tumors to lungs.[30] Therefore, experiments described in the "section

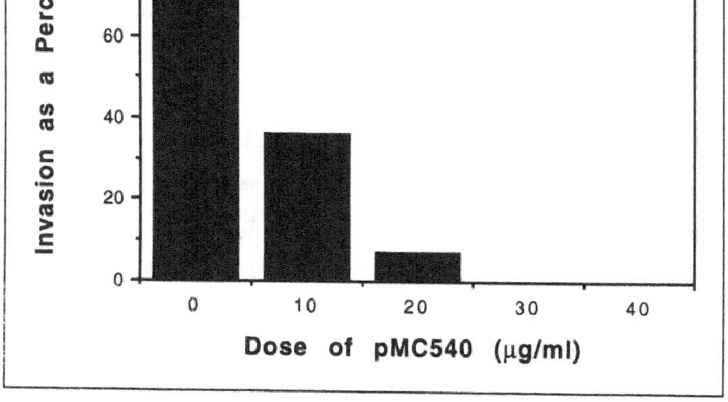

Fig. 4.11. Effect of pMC540 on the in vitro inhibition of HT-1080 human fibrosarcoma cell invasion through the reconstituted basement membranes. Results of a preliminary experiments are shown. Reprinted with permission from In Vivo 1995; 9: 103-108.

treatment of estrogen receptor negative established human breast tumor xenografts" were carried one step further. At the end of the experiment, autopsies of tumor bearing nude mice in the treated and control groups were performed. Examination of lungs from these groups revealed that the proportion of large tumors in the lungs of mice treated with either pMC540 or merodantoin was reduced as compared to the control groups. However, this reduction was statistically insignificant ($p > 0.5$) when total number of tumor foci were compared. These results suggest that pMC540 and merodantoin were not effective in preventing the metastasis of estrogen negative MDA-MB-435 tumors at the doses and schedule of injections employed. However, it is very important to note that the dose of pMC540 (250 mg/kg) or merodantoin (75 mg/kg), used in the treatment of breast tumors described in this book, was arbitrarily chosen. Our more recent studies have revealed that merodantoin is easily tolerated up to a dose of 500 mg/kg. In view of this information, it is not too unrealistic to predict that a significant improvement over the already very promising results could be made by employing the optimized doses and schedule of drug injections. Therefore, studies of the optimization of drug dose and schedule of drug injections are planned for a more complete exploitation of these agents.

COMBINED THERAPY OF BREAST TUMORS WITH RADIATION PLUS MERODANTOIN

It is well established now that the hypoxic cells present in solid tumors are believed to limit the success of radiotherapy[31,32] and perhaps even chemotherapy.[33] Over the years, a variety of methods such as hyperbaric oxygen, high linear energy transfer radiation, nitroheterocyclic radiosensitizers, hypoxic cell cytotoxins and oxygen carrying blood substitutes have been developed to counter the hypoxic cell problem.[34] Hypoxic radioresistance in tumors was first postulated in 1953,[35] and the histologic evidence was presented in 1955.[36] It was proposed that the vasculature in tumors is inadequate to provide sufficient nutrients and oxygen to all the cells in the tumor. Later, another hypothesis was advanced which suggested that hypoxia may arise due to fluctuations in blood flow caused by collapsed blood vessels when a region of tumor receives less oxygen for a period of time.[37] Indeed hypoxic cells now have been shown to exist in virtually all murine tumors and in several human tumors.[38,39] To date, most single therapeutic approaches have not been very effective against most cancer, in man. Thus, different modalities are generally combined in an effort to produce a more effective control or treatment of tumors. A most commonly used combination of modalities is chemotherapy plus radiotherapy or a combination of two or more chemotherapeutic agents. To enhance the effectiveness of solid tumor radiotherapy, two chemical approaches are considered. The first one is the pre-irradiation injection of radioprotective drugs, such as WR-2721, which selectively protects normal tissues and thereby allows the use of large radiation doses to the tumor.[40] The second approach requires injection of radiosensitizing drugs, such as RO-07-0582, which at least preferentially express their action within the hypoxic fraction of the tumor.[41]

Since the mechanism of tumor cell kill induced by pMC540 and merodantoin (see chapter 5) is different than the mechanism induced by radiation, we thought that an attack on tumor cells by these two very different modalities might yield even more desirable results. Therefore, in preliminary experiments, breast tumors in nude mice (bearing established human MCF-7 breast tumors) were first irradiated with 100 rads (a dose titrated to only slow down the growth of tumors for about 2 weeks) and then chemotherapy with pMC540 (250 mg/kg) or merodantoin (75 mg/kg) was initiated as described in the preceeding sections of this chapter. Treatments were terminated after 20 injections given over a period of 40 days. Results from this first set of experiments revealed that the combination of merodantoin plus radiation appeared to have produced an enhanced tumor regression whereas a similar combination with pMC540 did not. Since the radiation dose used was barely sufficient to slow down the tumor growth for a period of 2 weeks, it is reasonable to extrapolate that a small increase in radiation dose yielding approximately 50% tumor kill, when combined with merodantoin, may yield more favorable results. As described earlier, the dose of merodantoin needs to be titrated. Alternatively, radiation or chemotherapy dose could be administered after tumor growth has been first arrested by either one of these modalities. These and several other combinations of these experiments are underway.

In summary, data presented show that: 1) systemically injected preactivated compounds were easily tolerated in vivo models used;

2) they were effective against solid human breast tumor xenografts and 3) they show strong promise for the treatment of viral infections such as Herpes simplex, FeLV, SIV and HIV, demonstrating the potential clinical utility of these novel compounds.

REFERENCES

1. Pervaiz S, Battaglino M, Matthews JL et al. Biodistribution and toxicity of photoproducts of merocyanine 540. Cancer Chemother Pharmacol 1993; 31:467-74.
2. Roasli SB. Enzyme tests in diseases of the liver and hepatobiliary tract. In: Wilkinon J H, ed. The Principles and Practice of Diagnostic Enzymology. Chicago: Year Book, 1976:3030-39.
3. Podolsky DK, Isselbacher KJ. Diagnostic procedures in liver disease. In: Harrison's Principles of Internal Medicine. New York: McGraw-Hill, 1987:1315-21.
4. Kahler S. Immunodeficiency syndrome makes cats desirable HIV model. J Amer Vet Med Assoc 1992; 20:1674-75.
5. Wiggs RB, Lobprise HB, Matthews JL et al. Effects of preactivated MC540 in the treatment of lymphocytic plasmacytic stomatitis in feline leukemia virus and feline immunodeficiecy virus positive cats. J Veterinary Dentistry 1993; 10:9-13.
6. Friedman MA. New directions for breast cancer therapeutic research. Hematol. Oncol. Clin. of North Amer 1994; 8:113-19.
7. Arbuck SG, Dorr A, Friedman MA. Paclitaxel (Taxol) in breast cancer. Hematol Oncol Clin of North Amer 1994; 8:121-38.
8. Mattern J, Bak M, Han EW, Volm M. Human tumor xenografts as model for drug testing. Cancer Metast Rev 1988; 7:263-74.
9. Rygaard J. History and pathology. In: Boven E, Winograd B, eds. The Nude Mouse in Oncology Research. Boca Raton: CRC Press, 1991:1-11.
10. Chang P, Pervaiz S, Battaglino M et al. Synergy between preactivated photofrin-II and tamoxifen in killing retrofibroma, pseudomyxoma and breast cancer cells. Eur J Cancer 1991; 27:1034-39.
11. Patterson JS. "Novaldex" (tamoxifen) as an anticancer agent in humans. In: NonSteroidal Antiestrogens. Sydney: Academic Press, 1981:453-72.
12. Patterson JS, Battersby LA. Tamoxifen: an overview of recent studies in the field of oncology. Cancer Treat Rep. 1980; 64:775-78.
13. Shafie SM, Grantham FH. Role of hormones in the growth and regression of human breast cancer cells (MCF-7) transplanted into athymic mice. J Natl Cancer Inst 1981; 67:51–56.
14. Huseby RA, Maloney TM, McGrath CM. Evidence for a direct growth-stimulating effect of estradiol on human MCF-7 cells in vivo. Cancer Res 1984; 44:2654–59.
15. Gottardis MM, Robinson SP, Jordan VC. Estradiol-stimulated growth of MCF-7 tumors implanted in athymic mice: a model to

study the tumoristatic action of tamoxifen. J Steroid Biochem Mol Biol 1988; 20:311-14.
16. Iino Y, Wolf DM, Langan-Fahey SM et al. Reversible control of oestradiol-stimulated growth of MCF-7 tumors by tamifoxen in the athymic mouse. Br J Cancer 1991; 64:1019-24.
17. Satyaswaroop PG, Zaino RJ, Mortel R. Estrogen-like effects of tamoxifen on human endometrial carcinoma transplanted into nude mice. Cancer Res 1984; 44:4006-10.
18. Furr BJA, Jordan VC. The pharmacology and clinical uses of tamoxifen. Pharmacol Ther 1984; 25:127-205.
19. Fidler IJ, Gersten DM, Hart IR. The biology of cancer invasion and metastasis. Adv Cancer Res 1978; 28:149-250.
20. Fidler IJ. Tumor heterogeneity and the biology of cancer invasion and metastasis. Cancer Res 1979; 38:2651-60.
21. Poste G, Fidler IJ. The pathogenesis of cancer metastasis. Nature 1980; 283:139-46.
22. Nicolson GL. Cancer metastasis: tumor cell and host organ properties important in metastasis to specific secondary sites. Biochem Biophys Acta 1988; 948:175-24.
23. Liotta LA, Rao CN, Barsky SH. Tumor invasion and the extracellular matrix. Lab Invest 1983; 49:636-49.
24. Liotta LA, Rao CN, Wewer UM. Biochemical interactions of tumor cells with the basement membrane. Annu Rev Biochem 1986; 55:1037-57.
25. Humphries MJ, Olden K, Yamada KM. A synthetic peptide from fibronectin inhibits experimental metastasis of murine melanoma cells. Science 1987; 233:467-70.
26. Reich R, Thompson EW, Iwamoto Y et al. Effects of inhibitors of plasminogen activator, serine proteinases, and collagenase IV on the invasion of basement membranes by metastatic cells. Cancer Res 1988; 48:3307-12.
27. Alvarez OA, Carmichael DF, DeClerck YA. Inhibition of collagenolytic activity and metastasis of tumor cells by recombinant human tissue inhibitor of metyalloproteases. J Natl Cancer Inst 1990; 82:589-95.
28. Gehlsen KR, Argraves WS, Pierschbacher MD et al. Inhibition of in vitro tumor invasion by Arg-Gly-Asp-containing synthetic peptides. J Cell Biol 1988; 106:925-30.
29. Kumagai H, Tajima M, Ueno Y et al. Effect of cyclic RGD peptide on cell adhesion and tumor metastasis. Biochem Biophys Res Commun 1991; 177:74-82.
30. Bitonti Aj, Dumont JA, Bush TL et al. Regression of human breast tumor xenografts in response to (E)-2'-Deoxy-2' (fluoromethylene) cytidine, an inhibitor of ribonucleoside diphosphate reductase. Cancer Res 1994; 54:1485-90.
31. Bush RS, Jenkin RDT, Allt W et al. Definitive evidence for hypoxic cells influencing cure in cancer therapy. Br J Cancer 1978; 37:302-6.

32. Gatenby RA, Kessler HB, Rosenblum JS et al. Oxygen distribution in squamous cell carcinoma metastases: relationship to outcome of radiation therapy. Int J Radiat Oncol Biol Phys 1988; 14:831-38.
33. Tannock I. Response of aerobic and hypoxic cells in a solid tumor to adriamycin and cyclophosphamide and interaction of the drugs with radiation. Cancer Res 1982; 42:4921-26.
34. Coleman CN. Hypoxia in tumors: a paradigm for the approach to biochemical and physiological heterogeniety. J Natl Cancer Inst 1988; 80:310-17.
35. Gray LH, Conger AD, Ebert M. The concentration of oxygen dissolved in tissues at the time of radiation as a factor of radiotherapy. Br J Radiol 1953; 26:638-48.
36. Thomlinso RH, Gray LH. The histological structure of some human lung cancer and the possible implications for radiotherapy. Br J Cancer 1955; 9:539-49.
37. Brown JM. Evidence for acutely hypoxic cells in mouse tumors and a possible mechanism of reoxygenation. Br J Radiol 1979; 52:650-55.
38. Moulder JE, Rockwell S. Hypoxic fractions of solid tumors: experimental techniques, methods of analysis and a survey of existing data. Int J Radiat Oncol Biol Phys 1984; 10:695-12.
39. Carter DB, Silver IA. Quantitative measurements of oxygen tension in normal tissues and in tumor of patients before and after radiotherapy. Acta Radiol 1960; 53:233-56.
40. Yuhas JM, Storer JB. Differential chemoprotection of normal and malignant tissues. J Natl Cancer Inst 1969; 42:331-35.
41. Denekamp J, Harris SR. Tests of two electron affinic radiosensitizers in vivo using regrowth of an experimental carcinoma. Radiat Res 1975; 61:191-203.

CHAPTER 5

The Role of Topoisomerases and Apoptosis in the Mechanism of Action of Preactivated Compounds

In this chapter a description of the experimental data obtained to enhance our understanding of the underlying mechanism of action of pMC540, merocil and merodantoin is provided. The first set of experiments was designed to assess the potential involvement of oxygen derived species in the pMC540 mediated cytotoxicity. The rationale for this approach, at the time, was based on the observations that the in vitro cytotoxicity profile of pMC540 paralleled the one observed during conventional photodynamic therapy with native MC540, a process known to involve reactive oxygen species. Therefore, involvement of reactive oxygen species was chosen as a first step towards investigating the potential mechanism of action of pMC540. A brief description of these studies is followed by a discussion of the data related to the involvement of topoisomerases, apoptosis, mitochondrial morphology and function in the observed cytotoxicity mediated by preactivated compounds.

BACKGROUND

The free radical field is a large, multidisciplinary research area.[1-5] The basic chemistry of superoxide and hydroxyl radicals was determined many years ago by radiation chemists. The outline of lipid peroxidation was elucidated by scientists at the British Rubber Producers' Association; combustion is a free radical reaction; and some of the most detailed chemical work on peroxidation and antioxidants has been carried out in the food industry and by polymer scientists. In 1954, Gersman and Gilbert proposed that most of the damaging effects of elevated oxygen concentration on living organisms could be attributed to the formation of free radicals.[5] However, until the discovery of enzyme superoxide dismutase in 1968, this idea did not elicit much interest from scientists and clinicians alike. Superoxide dismutase is a specific enzyme that catalytically removes superoxides. The pioneering work of McCord and Fridovich has led to many fundamental discoveries including the fact that phagocytes use superoxide and hydrogen peroxide to aid bacterial killing.[2,3]

Oxygen free radicals or free radicals have been broadly defined as any species capable of independent existence that contains one or more unpaired electrons. Molecular oxygen has two unpaired electrons and is a diradical but weakly reactive. The effect of sequential addition of electrons to molecular oxygen is shown in Figure 5.1. The addition of a single electron to the outer electron shell of molecular oxygen produces a superoxide radical (O_2^-). Superoxide anion is enzymatically or nonenzymatically dismutated to hydrogen peroxide (H_2O_2), a product of the second electron reduction of oxygen. The half-life of hydrogen peroxide is sufficiently long enough such that it can exist in extracellular or intracellular environment. Upon metal-catalyzed reduction, hydrogen peroxide is converted to hydroxyl radical (•OH). Because of its highly reactive nature as well as its ability to be formed wherever there is ferrous iron, hydroxyl radical has received proportionately greater interest. It is noteworthy that in general most of the extracellular and intracellular iron exists in oxidized or ferric form.

Other free radicals have been identified in organic chemical models. These free radicals include physiological electron acceptors, such as ubiquinone, iron-oxygen conjugates, trioxides, peroxyl radicals and long lived radicals from cigarette smoke and tar. Ionizing radiation also generates free radicals directly, and some drugs and toxins, notably paraquat and menadione, generate radicals by redox cycling. Some constitutive antioxidants, including tocopherol (vitamin E), ascorbate (vitamin C) and reduced gluthione (GSH), exist as radical intermediates after a single-electron reduction in the detoxification of more toxic organic radical molecules.

The molybdo-flavo-enzymes. e.g. aldehyde dehydrogenase and xanthine dehydrogenase / oxidase can also generate O_2^- via a single-electron reduction of oxygen. These enzymes are located in the plasma membrane and microsomal membranes and thus are the sites for the generation of oxygen free radicals. There are three major pathways through which the fate of O_2^- is determined. In the first pathway the O_2^- is reduced to H_2O_2 by superoxide dismutase which regulates superoxide at 10^{-11} M. Since this dismutation reaction occurs rapidly, it is thought to be of little biological significance. In the second pathway the O_2^- can be protonated to form perhydroxy radical at Pk 4.7-4.9 (Fig. 5.1). Hydroxy radical HO_2^- is highly reactive and can initiate lipid peroxidation. In the third pathway the O_2^- can act as a powerful

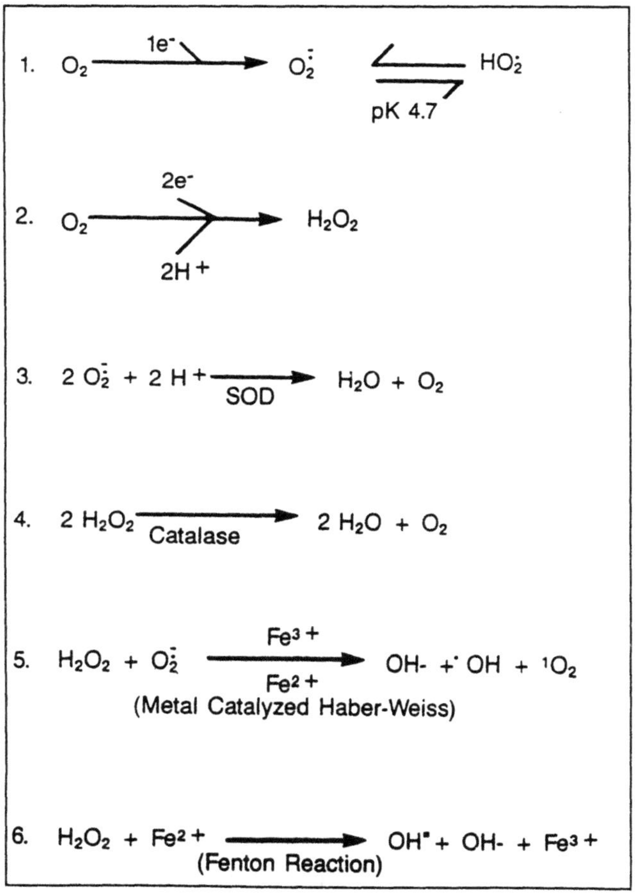

Fig. 5.1. Sequential addition of electrons to molecular oxygen.

reductant of metal ions including ferrous and ferric forms of iron, and thus recouples molecular oxygen.

As mentioned earlier, hydrogen peroxide can be generated enzymatically or nonenzymatically from superoxide radical. The enzymatic reaction is catalyzed by superoxide dismutase. Cytosolic fraction contains copper-zinc superoxide dismutase as the prevalent species, whereas manganese superoxide dismutase is predominantly present in mitochondrial membranes. The nonenzymatic hydrogen peroxide production occurs from three sources: superoxide, superoxide radical or the decomposition of peroxycytochrome P450 within the microsomal cytochrome P450 system, and the nonenzymatic reduction of hydroperoxy organic radicals by GSH. There are two mechanisms by which hydrogen peroxide is generated by peroxisomes: 1) internal flavin oxidases, fatty acid β–oxidases and α-hydroxyacid oxidases that generate superoxide radical; 2) membrane-bound enzymes, including xanthine oxidase capable of generating oxygen radicals. Within peroxisomes, hydrogen peroxide undergoes catalase-catalyzed oxidation/reduction to oxygen and water and is regulated at 10^{-8} to 10^{-9} M. Since oxygen and organic radicals are generated intracellularly and extracellularly, and hydrogen peroxide is known to diffuse freely across membranes and cells, this form of reduced oxygen could act as a reservoir for the generation of more toxic species. Hydrogen peroxide is also a substrate for myeloperoxidase, which catalyzes the reaction of hydrogen peroxide to form hypohalous acids and water. Hydrogen peroxide can also react with Cl^- to form hypochlorous acid, which can react with either amino acids or protein. Hypochlorous acid can chemically alter proteins. Hydrogen peroxide is also formed from two superoxide radicals. A hydroxyl radical can also be formed when a ferric ion is reduced to the ferrous state and hydrogen peroxide is then reduced, either by the Haber-Weiss reaction or the superoxide driven Fenton reaction.

Most complex organic molecules are susceptible to damage by reactive species such as hydroxyl radical (•OH). Hydroxyl radical is highly reactive and it can oxidize a target within three to five molecular radii. Any free radical that can extract a hydrogen atom will initiate lipid peroxidation. Thus hydroxyl radical or stable hydroperoxides (LOOH, formed by combination of two protons abstracted from polyunsaturated fatty acid molecules) can initiate lipid peroxidation while oxygen and hydrogen peroxide do not.

The highly electrophilic hydroxyl radical reacts with virtually any organic compound. It adds a hydroxyl group to aromatic compounds such as certain amino acids. In addition, sulfhydryl groups on amino acids can be oxidized to disulfide bridges, inactivating enzymes or destroying their catalytic sites. Hydroxyl radical can react to cleave DNA when it reacts with sugar moieties. The anticancer activity of adriamycin and daunorubicin is attributed to their ability to chelate iron and generate hydroxyl radicals. A large body of literature is easily available on the subject of reactive oxygen species and thus only a brief description is provided.

INVOLVEMENT OF REACTIVE OXYGEN SPECIES IN THE CYTOTOXIC ACTION MEDIATED BY pMC540

As stated earlier, the cytotoxicity profile of pMC540 resembles the one obtained during the conventional photodynamic therapy with native MC540. The process of photodynamic therapy is known to involve reactive oxygen species. In addition, one peak in the reverse phase HPLC elution profile of pMC540 was suspected to correspond with the presence of hydroperoxides. Thus, pMC540 (Chapter 2) was first analyzed for the presence of hydroperoxides species as described below.

For the analysis of hydroperoxide species, freshly prepared pMC540 was analyzed by using a hemoglobin catalyzed reaction of the hydroperoxides with 10-N-methylcarbamoyl-3,7-dimethylamino-10-H-phenothiazine. This reaction produces a stoichiometric quantity of methylene blue, which can be quantified by absorption spectroscopic detection at 675 nm.[6] Results from this assay clearly showed (Table 5.1) that a significant amount (27.4 nmol/ml) of hydroperoxides were present in pMC540 as compared to the extremely low levels (0-1.5 nmol/ml) of hydroperoxides present in the unactivated compound.[7] A strong correlation ($r = .93$) between the levels of hydroperoxides and percent of tumor cell kill upon exposure to pMC540 was also observed (Table 5.2). However, upon storage for seven days, there was a significant (70%) loss of detectable hydroperoxides and a concomitant loss in observed cytotoxicity. The hydroperoxides formed may be due to the oxidation of the MC540 molecule at ground state by a molecule of singlet oxygen generated at triplet state.

It is now well established that primary, secondary and tertiary structures of proteins are altered upon exposure to hydroxyl (•OH) and superoxides.[8-10] In view of our observation that treatment of HIV-1 with pMC540 inhibits its binding to the target cells (discussed in chapter 2), we thought that perhaps some structure(s) such as gp120 on the surface of HIV-1 might be susceptible to the action of pMC540. To investigate this possibility, we first elected to study the effects of pMC540 on bovine serum albumin (BSA), a well-characterized, easily available and inexpensive protein. Our data demonstrated that exposure of BSA to pMC540 caused a rapid loss of native tryptophan fluorescence (Table 5.3). These results were interpreted to suggest that hydroxyl or superoxide species in pMC540 may have caused loss of tryptophan.[4] However, loss of tryptophan residues could not be quantified because tryptophan residues are destroyed upon hydrolysis of the sample for amino acid analysis.

In an attempt to obtain a more definitive answer, free L-tryptophan was treated with pMC540 and its fluorescence was measured. However, free L-tryptophan did not appear to be affected

Table 5.1. Determination of hydroperoxides in pMC540

Cytotoxicity	Absorbance (675 nm)	Concentration (nmol/ml)	Amount of Peroxide (nmol/ml)	Percent Toxicity %
Purified water (control)	0.001	–	–	–
10% Ethanol [solvent control (blank)]	0.008	–	–	–
Cumene hydroperoxide (standard)	0.132	–	–	–
Nonactivated MC540	0.004	56.45	0.0	–
pMC540 (fresh)	0.076	56.45	27.42	88.0
*pMC540 (stored at RT for 4 months)	0.000	56.45	–	0.0

*pMC540 loses its cytotoxicity after storage at room temperature for nine days. Results shown are that of a representative experiment repeated once with < 10% variability. Reprinted with permission from Free Radical Biology and Medicine 1992; 12:389-396.

by the treatment with pMC540. In view of these findings, we proposed that one possible explanation of these observations could be that amino acids may have to be in the native configuration of the protein for pMC540 to mediate its effect. Further evidence of the involvement of hydroxyl species was obtained by examining the bityrosine production which is a useful marker for protein modification by hydroxyl radical.[11] However, treatment of BSA with pMC540 did not result in the production of bityrosine (Table 5.4). It is important to note that certain reactive oxygen species, e.g. superoxides, can inhibit the formation of bityrosine by re-reduction of tyrosyl radicals.[12] One mechanism of protein aggregation involves the formation of intermolecular bityrosine formation. Protein aggregates were not seen by the SDS-PAGE analysis of BSA treated with pMC540, confirming the absence of bityrosine formation. However, fragmentation products of pMC540 treated BSA were detected by SDS-PAGE analysis. These products are known

Table 5.2. Correlation of cytotoxicity with the amount of hydroperoxides in pMC540

Days After Preactivation	Amount of Peroxide (nmol/ml)	Cytotoxicity* %
0	12.99 ± 0.06	55.6 ± 1.1
1	10.24 ± 0.99	36.9 ± 8.4
2	9.84 ± 0.06	37.4 ± 5.2
6	11.02 ± 0.99	37.4 ± 5.2
7	9.06 ± 0.04	35.4 ± 4.5
8	5.90 ± 0.16	14.3 ± 0.5

*For cytotoxicity determinations, Daudi cells (5×10^5 cells/ml) were treated with 80 mg/ml of pMC540. Coefficient of correlation (r = 0.93) was calculated by linear regression analysis. Mean ± S.E.M. of three separate experiments are shown. Reprinted with permission from Free Radical Biology and Medicine 1992; 12:389-396.

Table 5.3. Amino acid modification by pMC540

Tryptophan Oxidation	
Samples	**Relative Fluorescence λ_{ex} = 280, λ_{em} = 345**
1. PBS	0.75 ± 0.5
2. BSA (0.5 mg/ml)	65.63 ± 12.63
3. pMC540 (1 mg/ml)	0.63 ± 0.48
4. BSA (0.5 mg/ml) + pMC540 (0.5 mg/ml)	0.88 ± 0.63
5. BSA (0.5 mg/ml) + pMC540 (1 mg/ml)	0.312 ± 0.24

Reprinted with permission from Free Radical Biology and Medicine 1992; 12:389-396.

to be produced by the combined action of more than one reactive oxygen species (for example, •OH + O_2^-).[9] Thus, observed results could mean that more than one reactive oxygen species may be involved in the biological activity of pMC540. However, the mechanism of protein fragmentation does not appear to involve peptide bond hydrolysis because free amino groups were not detected (Table 5.5) by fluorescamine which reacts with free amino groups to form a fluorescent product that can be measured spectrophotometrically.[13]

Amino acid analysis of BSA treated with pMC540 shows (Table 5.6) loss of several amino acid residues where tyrosine residues appear to be most affected. However, it is at best very difficult to deduce the probable nature of the oxidant from amino acid analysis data. The findings that treatment with pMC540 causes protein fragmentation and loss of several amino acid residues could be used to speculate that HIV-1 surface proteins might be affected by this agent in a similar manner. However, lack of homology between HIV-1 surface proteins and BSA could not be used in support of this argument. Nonetheless, this hypothesis remains to be tested.

Table 5.4. Bityrosine formation

Samples	Relative Fluorescence λ_{ex} = 325, λ_{em} = 415
1. PBS	0.5 ± 0.00
2. BSA (0.5 mg/ml)	8.17 ± 0.29
3. pMC540 (1 mg/ml)	1.00 ± 0.50
4. BSA (0.5 mg/ml) + pMC540 (1 mg/ml)	8.17 ± 0.29

BSA (0.5 mg) was incubated for 2 hours with 0.5 mg/ml and 1.0 mg/ml of pMC540 at 37°C. Tryptophan oxidation was studied at 280 nm excitation and 345 nm emission. Bityrosine production was determined by measuring the fluorescence at 415 nm of samples excited at 325 nm. Results are mean ± S.D. of three separate sets of experiments. Reprinted with permission from Free Radical Biology and Medicine 1992; 12:389-396.

Table 5.5. Peptide hydrolysis by pMC540

Samples	Relative Fluorescence λ_{ex} = 390, λ_{em} = 475
1. PBS	0.75 ± 0.35
2. BSA (0.5 mg/ml)	10.75 ± 0.35
3. pMC540 (1 mg/ml)	7.00 ± 0.71
4. BSA (0.5 mg/ml) + pMC540 (1 mg/ml)	7.50 ± 0.71

BSA (0.5 mg) was treated with 0.5 mg and 1 mg/ml of pMC540 for 2 hours. Peptide hydrolysis was studied by fluorescamine reactivity. Fluorescence was measured with a Perkin Elmer spectrofluorometer, Model 204-A. Data shown are mean ± S.D. of three separate sets of experiments. Reprinted with permission from Free Radical Biology and Medicine 1992; 12:389-396.

While the data presented implicate the involvement of more than one reactive oxygen species, at least in part, a conclusive case clearly demonstrating the involvement of reactive oxygen species could not be made. Since at the time these studies were carried out, the chemical identity of the individual photoproducts in pMC540 was not known, this paucity of information added to the tentativeness of the foregoing conclusion. Later, when three photoproducts, merocil, meroxazole and merodantoin were isolated and chemically characterized, the studies of the mechanism of action were expanded by further investigating the role of reactive oxygen species in the observed cytotoxicity.

Effect of Scavengers, Antioxidants and Metal Chelators

In this study the effect of hydroxyl radical scavengers, antioxidant enzymes and iron chelators on the photoproduct treated Daudi lymphoma cells was investigated. Cytotoxicity studies revealed that meroxazole was virtually nontoxic to cultured tumor cells. Therefore, all subsequent studies were carried out using pMC540, merocil and merodantoin. Experiments were performed to determine whether pMC540, merocil or merodantoin produce hydroxyl radicals in the manner of the anticancer drugs quinone and menadione, which are known to function as electron acceptors and then produce hydroxyl radicals by reduction of oxygen molecules.[14,15] Results show (Table 5.7) that only pMC540-mediated cytotoxicity was suppressed in the presence of catalase but not in the presence

Table 5.6. Amino acid analysis of untreated and pMC540 treated bovine serum albumin

Amino Acid	BSA	BSA*
ASX	58.86	60.48
THR	33.32	32.48
SER	24.51	25.37
GLX	88.47	88.96
PRO	0.00	0.00
GLY	17.64	18.65
ALA	51.51	51.95
C as 1/2CYS	5.25	3.39
VAL	36.85	32.38
MET	4.27	4.34
ILE	14.13	11.99
LEU	66.91	65.87
TYR	20.54	14.89
PHE	28.97	27.81
HIS	17.65	19.13
LYS	56.44	57.15
TRP	0.00	0.01
ARG	22.46	22.67

*0.5 BSA treated with 1 mg pMC540; Values are reported as residues per mole. Reprinted with permission from Free Radical Biology and Medicine 1992; 12:389-396.

of superoxide dismutase (SOD) or diethylenetriamine pentacetic acid (DETAPAC). All of these agents are known to be incapable of penetrating the cell membrane.[16] However, iron chelator, bipyridine, enters cells freely.[17] In the presence of bipyridine, the pMC540-, merocil- and merodantoin-mediated cytotoxicity was significantly suppressed. These data suggested that the site of interaction between iron and the novel compounds may be intracellular. Since H_2O_2 is freely permeable across cell membranes, the slight protective effect of exogenous catalase could result from a reduction in the intracellular peroxide concentration by the extracellular

Table 5.7. Effect of reactive oxygen scavengers on Daudi cell susceptibility to pMC540, merocil and merodantoin

Agent	Function	Concentration	pMC540 % cell kill (mean ± SD)	Merocil % cell kill (mean ± SD)	Merodantoin % cell kill (mean ± SD)
None			89.3 ± 2.51	93.0 ± 5.56	86.0 ± 4.24
Catalase	Hydrogen peroxide scavenger	750 units/mL	40.0 ± 1.00*	91.66 ± 2.88	90.5 ±0.71
SOD	Superoxide anion scavenger	1.25 µg/mL	84.0 ± 2.82	95.0 ± 1.00	ND
SOD + Catalase	Inhibition of hydroxyl radical generation	0.63 µg/mL + 325 units/mL	61.0 ± 2.80*	96.0 ± 1.41	82.0 ± 8.90
Mannitol	Hydroxyl radical scavenger	20 mM	87.50 ± 3.53	98.0 ± 1.40	85.50 ± 3.53
DMSO	Hydroxyl radical scavenger	400 mM	87.0 ± 1.7	92.5 ± 3.53	87.0 ± 2.90
Bipyridine	Iron chelator	60 µM	31.66 ± 5.13* (p = .0001)	72.0 ± 4.73* (p = .0012)	62.33 ± 6.43 (p = .0008)
DETAPAC	Iron chelator	60 mM	90.0 ± 1.14	93.0 ± 1.0	79.0 ± 1.10

SOD indicates superoxide dismutase; ND, not done; DMSO, dimethyl sulfoxide; and DETAPAC, diethylenetriamine pentacetic acid. Daudi cells (1 x 10^6 cells/ml) were treated with different compounds in the presence of reactive oxygen scavengers at indicated concentrations. After overnight incubation, percent cell kill was determined by trypan blue dye exclusion test.

enzyme. Superoxide anion in itself does not easily cross the tumor cell membrane. Taken together this scenario may explain the observed ineffectiveness of SOD.

Results with DETAPAC and bipyridine also suggest that either the iron-catalyzed Haber-Weiss reaction[18] or, in the presence of iron, a direct interaction between the novel compounds and H_2O_2 may result in the formation of hydroxyl radical,[19] which could explain the findings with these compounds. Clearly, these data do not provide a strong evidence for the involvement of reactive oxygen species in pMC540 mediated cytotoxicity. Irrespective of the precise mechanism involved, the oxidizing power of •OH radical[20] could exert a powerful oxidant stress at multiple cellular sites in tumor cells treated with the drugs that produce them. In summary, while the involvement of reactive oxygen species in the observed cytotoxicity induced by pMC540, merocil and merodantoin is likely, they do not appear to play a predominant role, and thus involvement of other potential mechanisms described below were also considered.

During the course of the studies described above, we were also evaluating the efficacy of preactivated compounds against a panel of breast cancer cell lines. One human breast cancer cell line MDA-MB-231 turned out to be particularly resistant to the cytotoxic action of pMC540 and its chemically synthesized isolates merocil and merodantoin. This was unusual because other estrogen receptor positive and estrogen receptor negative breast cancer cell lines such as MCF-7, BT-20 and T47D were quite susceptible to the cytotoxic action of these agents. The question was why this particular breast cancer cell line was so resistant while others were not? Based on very well known facts regarding multidrug resistance to chemotherapeutic drugs, a hypothesis consisting of the following possibilities was advanced. We speculated that resistance to these compounds may be due to expression of multidrug resistance phenotype by MDA-MB-231 cells; or topoisomerases may be involved since many anticancer drugs mediate their effect via the involvement of topoisomerases. Therefore, a systematic investigation of these possibilities was initiated.

TOPOISOMERASES

Most cytotoxic compounds with significant antitumor activity can be assigned to one of two categories. The first category includes those compounds or treatments that antagonize DNA metabolism in some way; for example, by interfering with the biosynthesis of DNA precursors (Methotrexate) or by damaging the DNA directly (ionizing radiation, alkylating agents). The second category includes compounds such as vinca alkaloids, that disrupt critical cellular structures by interfering with tubulin formation (Taxol and Texotere). Acridines and epipodophyllotoxins were also found to interact with the intracellular target DNA topoisomerase II.[21, 22]

More recently another anti-neoplastic compound, Campothecin, was found to inhibit DNA topoisomerase I in cells.[23] Campothecin I[24] was first isolated from the wood, bark, and fruits of *Camptotheca acuminata* Decaisne (Nyssaceae). The interesting manner in which the seeds of this Chinese tree were collected from Szechwan, Yunnan, and Kwangsi provinces and brought to the United States many years ago has been reported.[25] Campothecin, an alkaloid, causes a high degree of inhibition in the growth of L1210 leukemia and solid tumors in rodents.[26-28] However, in clinical trials it proved to be ineffective. Much later it was realized that the sodium salt of campothecin used in clinical trials is only about one tenth as potent as the parent compound.[29]

It was demonstrated that the inhibitors of enzymes topoisomerase I and II also possess antitumor activity. Later these enzymes were identified immunologically as relevant drug targets. To date, clinically useful topoisomerase inhibitors are known to kill tumor cells but only with modest selectivity because in patients treated with such drugs significant toxicities occurred as a result of this treatment. The cell killing can be modulated with qualitative or quantitative alterations in topoisomerase I[30,31] or topoisomerase II.[32,33]

Topoisomerase II is known primarily for its enzymatic role in the regulation of the topology of supercoiled DNA. Several cellular functions such as replication, transcription, recombination, repair, chromosome condensation and disjunction are dependent on the topological interconversions.[34-36] DNA topoisomerase II transiently breaks and then reseals the DNA helix, altering DNA linking number and allowing adjustment of topology. In vitro experiments have revealed that when topoisomerase II and DNA are mixed, a cleavage and relegation equilibrium is established. Enzyme induced cleavage products are isolated by the addition of sodium dodecyl sulfate and proteinase K to the reaction mixture.

The function of sodium dodecyl sulfate and proteinase K is not clear and their action may either denature and trap existing complex or induce DNA cleavage within an existing precleavage DNA-topoisomerase II complex. In any event, the product of this enzymatic activity is a covalent topoisomerase II-DNA complex in which the enzyme is attached to the 4 base protruding 5' termini of the cleaved member [37,38] via an O^4-phosphotyrosyl bond.[39]

Another feature of the DNA-topoisomerase II reaction is that ATP, which acts as a cofactor for the enzyme's DNA strand passage reaction, is not required for cleavage activity.[34-36] However the reaction is absolutely dependent on the presence of preferably magnesium or other divalent cations. Yet another feature of DNA-topoisomerase II reaction is that there is an equilibrium between DNA cleavage and relegation, which could be shifted towards relegation by the addition of salts.[38-40] The relegation portion of the DNA cleavage-relegation reaction can be separated by using an in vitro assay which allows examination of the kinetics of the reaction without the cleavage activity as well as the mechanism of action of anticancer drugs.[40] Such experiments have revealed that topoisomerase II reaction appears to produce double-stranded breaks in DNA by making two sequential single stranded cuts in the DNA strands.

Drugs that interact with the enzyme topoisomerase II have been found to be particularly useful in the chemotherapeutic treatment of certain cancers.[41-43] Both intercalative and nonintercalative anticancer drugs appear to stabilize, at least in part, the enzyme-DNA cleavage complex.

INTERACTION OF pMC540 AND MERODANTOIN WITH TOPOISOMERASE II

To determine the possible involvement of topoisomerases in the cytotoxicity induced by pMC540 and merodantoin, a topoisomerase II drug screening assay (TopoGen, Columbus, Ohio) was used. This assay allows the detection of two classes of topoisomerase inhibitors: those that stimulate formation of cleavable complexes and those that antagonize topoisomerase II action on the DNA. Treatment of cell free substrate DNA in the presence of human topoisomerase II with or without pMC540 or merodantoin was carried out. Results show that both pMC540 and merodantoin caused the formation of a cleavable complex (linear

DNA species). The yield of linear DNA species increased with the increasing concentration of pMC540 and merodantoin (Figure 5.2). The conversion of supercoiled DNA substrate (pRYG) was inhibited in the reaction that contained VM-26, an inhibitor of topoisomerase II. These data indicate that the activity of pMC540 and merodantoin was topoisomerase II dependent and that these compounds do not antagonize its action.[44]

As stated earlier, one estrogen receptor negative breast cancer cell line MDA-MB-231 was found to be particularly resistant (Table 5.8) to the cytotoxic action of these compounds while estrogen receptor positive MCF-7, T47D and several other cell lines were quite sensitive. We speculated that this resistance may be due to the expression of multidrug resistance (MDR) phenotype by MDA-MB-231 cells, or involvement of topoisomerases.

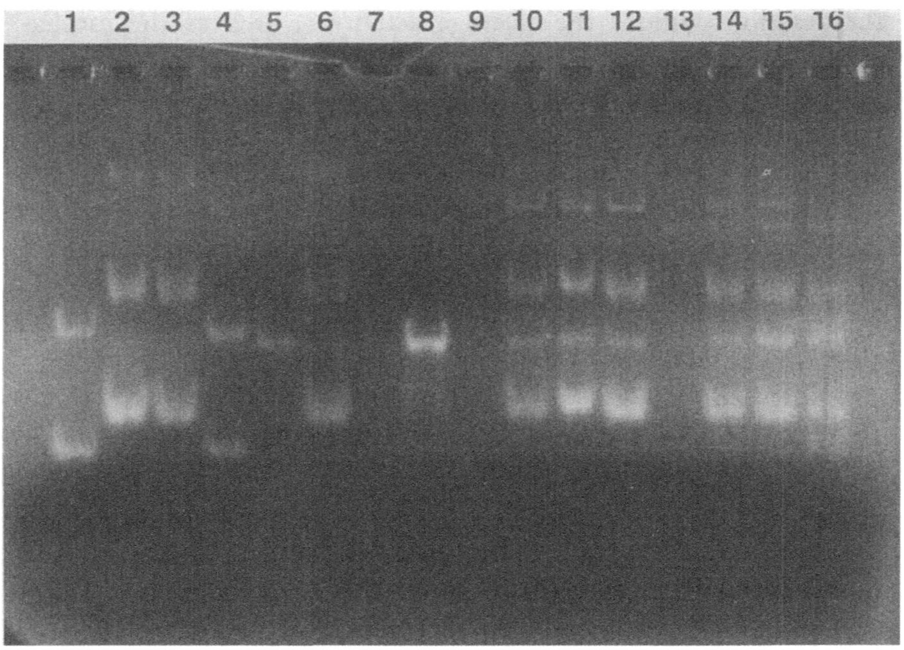

Fig. 5.2. Topoisomerase II dependent cleavage activity of pMC540 and merodantoin. Lane 1, pRYGDNA + Topo II (enzyme control), Lane 2, supercoiled DNA marker; Lane 3, solvent control (2.5% EtOH); Lane 4, solvent + Topo II; Lane 5, Linear DNA marker; Lane 6, supercoiled DNA in cleavage buffer; Lane 7, 9 and 13 blank; Lane 8, VM26 + Topo II; Lane 10–12, Topo II + pMC540 (70.2 μm, 140.4 μm and 210.6 μm); Lane 14–15, Topo II + merodantoin (51.6 μm, and 103.3 μm/ml); Lane 16, Topo II + DMSO (solvent used for merodantoin). Reprinted with permission from Anticancer Drugs 1994; 5:557-566.

Therefore, to determine whether the observed insensitivity of MDA-MB-231 cells to pMC540 and merodantoin was related to the expression of MDR phenotype, both MCF-7 and MDA-MB-231 cells were analyzed for *mdr1* gene amplification, over expression of the *mdr1* gene, and expression of P-glycoprotein. Amplification of *mdr1* gene was not detected by Southern blotting in these cell lines.[45] Over expression of mRNA of the *mdr1* gene was not detected, and Western blot using C219 monoclonal antibody was also negative for both cell lines. These data suggested that the involvement of multidrug resistance was unlikely, and the observed resistance to pMC540 and merodantoin cannot be explained by the involvement of MDR phenotype. However, there are other mechanisms of drug resistance that do not include P-glycoprotein. For example, a defective drug transport[46,47] or drug detoxification via the involvement of glutathione[48] or cross resistance to natural product drugs known to interfere with DNA topoisomerase II activity or a combination of more than one of these forms of resistance have been reported.[49,50] These alternative mechanisms for pMC540 or merodantoin have not been ruled out.

Table 5.8. Effect of pMC540 and merodantoin in MCF-7 and MDA-MB-231 breast cancer cells.

Treatment	Dose	Clonogenic Growth in MCF-7 (No. of colonies)	MDA-MB-231 (No. of colonies)
Untreated		214.3 ± 56.3	274.6 ± 2.1
pMC540	(70.2 µM for 24 h)	0.7 ± 8.6	273 ± 4.2
	(140.4 µM for 24 h)	0	170 ± 42.4
	(70.2 µM for 48 h)	0	270 ± 6.9
Merodantoin	(61.95 µM for 24 h)	1.3 ± 1.5	156 ± 7.2
	(103.25 µM for 24 h)	0	101 ± 9
	(61.95 µM for 48 h)	0	122 ± 54

Breast cancer cells (5×10^3 cell/25 cm^2 flask)were treated with indicated doses of pMC540 or merodantoin. After incubation for 24 or 48 hours cells were washed to remove the drugs and incubated in drug-free growth medium for a period of 14 days. Control flasks were seeded with 1×10^3 cells /flask. Colonies consisting of 50 or more cells were counted as clonogenic growth. Results of a representative experiment (mean ± S.D) performed in triplicate are shown.

CATALYTIC ACTIVITY OF TOPOISOMERASES FROM BREAST CANCER CELL LINES

Next, studies involving topoisomerase II were initiated to determine the relationship between DNA Topo II activity and pMC540 and merodantoin sensitive MCF-7, and insensitive MDA-MB-231 breast cancer cell lines.[45] First, the catalytic activity of Topo II obtained from cellular and nuclear extracts of breast cancer cells was determined by decatenation of the kDNA network.[51,52] Several experiments were carried out in which Topo II activity (concentration adjusted to equivalence) in crude nuclear and cellular extracts from MCF-7 and MDA-MB-231 was determined. These experiments revealed that Topo II activities were two- to three-fold lower in crude nuclear extracts from MDA-MB-231 than in extracts from MCF-7 cells, as could be seen by comparing band intensities of the minicircles in the serial dilutions (Fig. 5.3). The bands near the top of the gel were products of incompletely decatenated kDNA.[52] In crude cellular extracts from MDA-

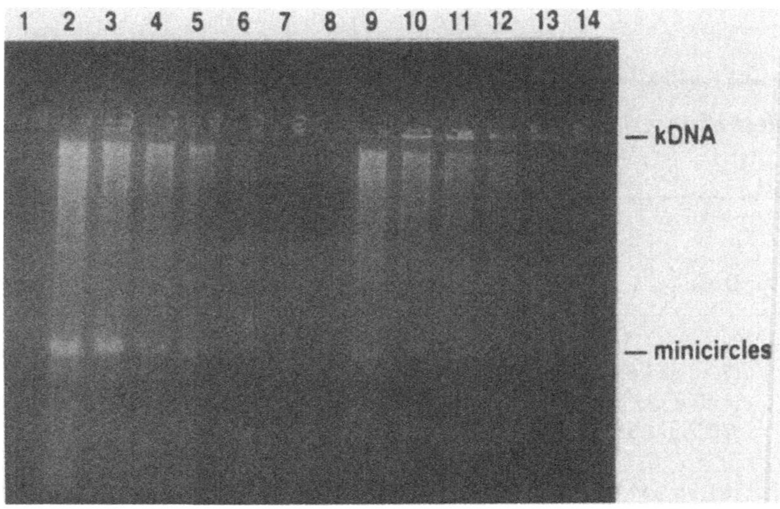

Fig. 5.3. Topoisomerase II activity in nuclear extracts from MCF-7 and MDA-MB-231. Topoisomerase II activity was monitored by the decatenation assay. Reaction mixture (25 µl) containing 2.0 µg of kDNA and various dilutions of nuclear extracts from MCF-7 (lanes 2–7) or MDA-MB-231 (lanes 9–14) and blank (lane 8) were incubated for 30 min at 37° C and analyzed. The extract protein amounts added were: control, no extract protein (lane 1), 2.5 µg (lanes 2 and 9), 1.25 µg (lanes 3 and 10), 0.625 µg (lanes 4 and 11), 0.313 µg (lanes 5 and 12), 0.156 µg (lanes 6 and 13), 0.078 µg (lanes 7 and 14). Reprinted with permission from Anti-Cancer Research 1995; 15:295-304.

MB-231, Topo II activities were undetectable. However, in the case of MCF-7, minicircles were detectable (Fig. 5.4). In the absence of ATP, decatenation of kDNA was undetectable, suggesting that Topo I was probably not involved. To further exclude the possibility that the decrease in Topo II activity in extracts from MDA-MB-231 was a nonspecific phenomenon, Topo I catalytic activities in the same extracts were also determined. Topo I activities in extracts from MCF-7 and MDA-MB-231 were compared by determining the highest dilution factor that was needed for the ATP-independent relaxation of all supercoiled pBR322 DNA.[53] The Topo I activities were almost identical in nuclear extracts (Fig. 5.5) and cellular extracts from both cell lines. The relaxation of supercoiled pBR322 was completely due to Topo I activity and not endonuclease activity in these extracts, because all of the newly formed relaxed circles appeared to be closed circles (as determined by gel electrophoresis) in the presence of ethidium bromide. The possibility that reduction in Topo II activity may be due to the differences in the growth kinetics of MCF-7 and

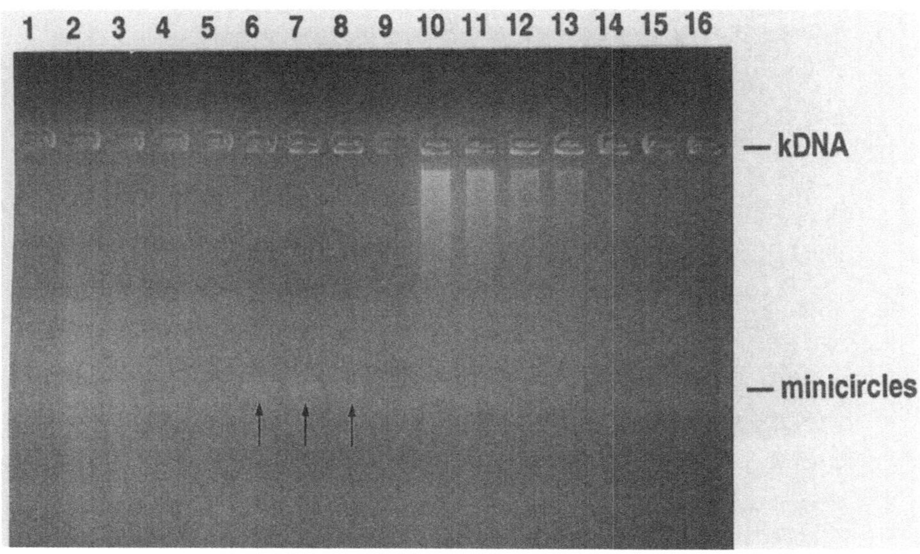

Fig. 5.4. Topoisomerase II activity in cellular extracts form MCF-7 and MDA-MB-231. Topoisomerase II activity in cellular extract from MCF-7 (lanes 2–8), MDA-MB-231 (lanes 10–16) and blank (lane 9) was monitored by the decatenation assay. The extract protein amounts added were: control, no extract protein (lane 1), 5 μg (lanes 2 and 10), 2.5 μg (lanes 3 and 11), 1.25 μg (lanes 4 and 12), 0.625 μg (lanes 5 and 13), 0.313 μg (lanes 6 and 14), 0.156 μg (lanes 7 and 15), 0.078 μg (lanes 8 and 16).

MDA-MB-231 cells was also considered and their doubling times were compared. This possibility was ruled out because the doubling time of MDA-MB-231 (43 hours) was only 3 hours less then the doubling time of MCF-7 cells.

DNA CLEAVAGE ACTIVITY

Whether the reduced Topo II activity in nuclear extracts from MDA-MB-231 has an effect on the pMC540- or merodantoin-induced formation of the cleavage complex was studied in an in vitro DNA cleavage assay using supercoiled pRYG and nuclear extract.[54-56] Both pMC540 and merodantoin stimulated the Topo II-mediated DNA cleavage in the presence of ATP and nuclear extracts, as shown in Figure 5.6 by the formation of linearized pRYG DNA (form III) after SDS proteinase K treatment. Increased linearized pRYG DNA was detectable in extracts from MCF-7 cells in the presence of pMC540 and merodantoin as compared to extracts from MDA-MB-231. This is probably due to decreased Topo

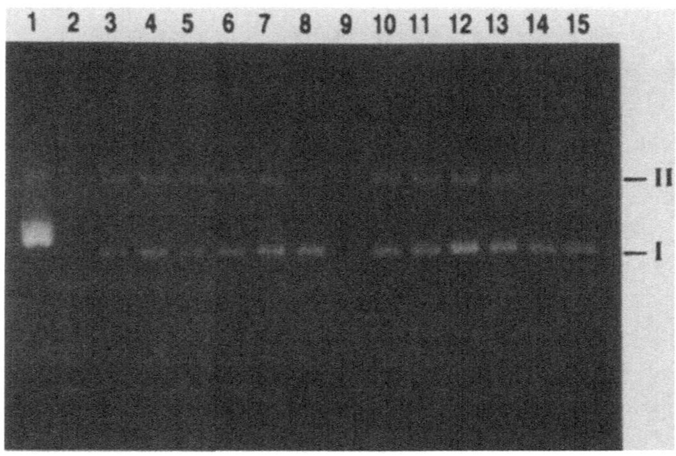

Fig. 5.5. Topoisomerase I activity in nuclear extracts from MCF-7 and MDA-MB-231. Reaction mixture (25 µl) containing 0.9 µg of supercoiled pBR322 and various dilutions of nuclear extracts from MCF-7 (lanes 3–8) or MDA-MB-231 (lanes 10–15) and blank (lanes 2 and 9) were incubated for 30 min at 37° C and analyzed. The extract protein amounts added were: control, no extract protein (lane 1), 1 µg (lanes 3 and 10), 0.5 µg (lanes 4 and 11),) 0. 25 µg (lanes 5 and 12), 0.125 µg (lanes 6 and 13), 0.0625 mg (lanes 7 and 14), 0.0313 µg (lanes 8 and 15). Reprinted with permission from Anti-Cancer Research 1995; 15:295-304.

II activity in MDA-MB-231. The addition of high salt (0.5 M NaCl) after pre-incubation with pMC540 and merodantoin (Fig. 5.7) reduced the DNA cleavage significantly in nuclear extracts from MCF-7 as well as MDA-MB-231, suggesting that these activities were Topo II mediated.[45]

WESTERN BLOT ANALYSIS OF TOPO II

The amount of 170 kD form of Topo II enzyme in nuclear extract and whole cell lysates of the three breast cancer cell lines (T47D, MDA-MB-231 and MCF-7) was determined by Western blot analysis (Fig. 5.8). Results of this experiment show that the Topo II present in the nuclear extract is representative of the Topo II present in the whole cell. These findings are supported by additional evidence obtained from immunoblot analysis of extracted nuclei and cytosolic fractions which revealed no detectable Topo II (170 kD) in the cytosolic fractions and only a very low level in extracted nuclei.[45] A similar comparison of Topo II levels (170

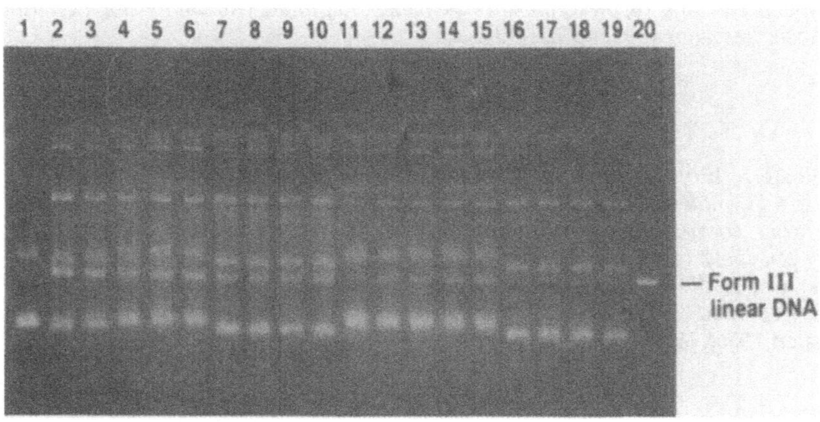

Fig. 5.6. pMC540 and merodantoin (MD) stimulated cleavage of pRYG DNA in the presence of nuclear extracts from MCF-7 and MDA-MB-231. DNA cleavage reactions were done as described earlier.[40] First various concentrations of pMC540 and MD were added to the reaction mixture (20 µl) containing 0.3 µg of supercoiled pRYG and then 2.5 µg of nuclear extract protein from MCF-7 (lanes 2-10) or MDA-MB-231 (lanes 11-19) was added. After 30 min. at 37°C, the reaction was terminated with SDS, proteinase K was added and DNA sample preparation was done as previously described.[40] Lane 1, control, no drug, no extract protein; lanes 2 and 11, no drug; lanes 3-6, 35.1, 70.2, 140.4 and 210.6 µM pMC540; lanes 7-10, 20.65, 41.3, 61.95, and 103.25 µM merodantoin; lanes 12-15 and lanes 16-19 same as lanes 3-6 and lanes 7-10 respectively. Lane 20, pRYG linear DNA marker. Reprinted with permission from Anti-Cancer Research 1995; 15:295-304.

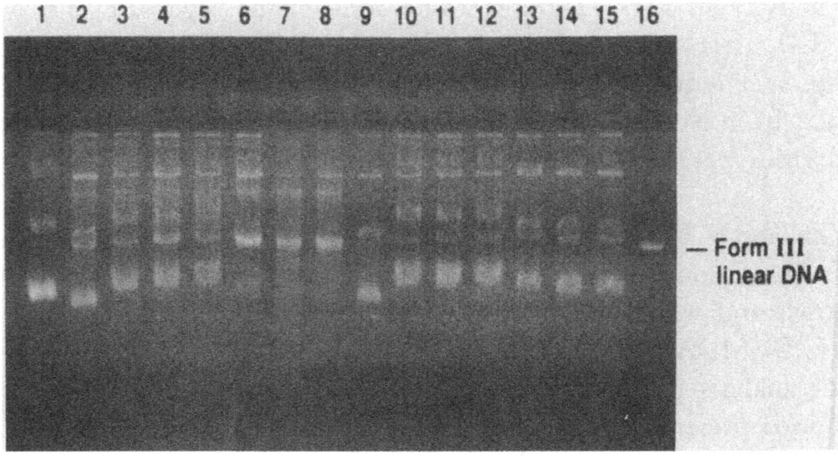

Fig. 5.7. Reversal of pMC540 and merodantoin induced DNA cleavage by high-salt treatment. The reaction mixture (20 µl) containing 0.3 µg of supercoiled pRYG and 2.5 µg of nuclear extract protein from MCF-7 (lanes 2–8) or MDA-MB-231 (lanes 9–15) was incubated at 37°C for 30 min. in the presence of 210.6 µM pMC540 and merodantoin (MD) 103.25 µM. 5 M NaCl was then added to the reaction mixture (0.5 M NaCl final). Termination of the reaction with SDS at various times after the second incubation, proteinase K treatment and sample preparation was done as previously described. Lane 1, control, no drug, no extract protein; lanes 2 and 9 control, no drug; lanes 3–5 pMC540; lanes 6–8 merodantoin, reactions were terminated at 0, 15 and 30 min. after the addition of NaCl; lanes 10–12 and lanes 13–15, same as lanes 3–5 and lanes 6–8 respectively. Lane 16, pRYG linear DNA marker. Reprinted with permission from Anti-Cancer Research 1995; 15:295-304.

Fig. 5.8. Western blot analysis of 170 kD topoisomerase II in whole cell lysates (150 µg total protein/lane from normal exponentially growing breast cancer cell lines); lane 1, 170 kD molecular weight marker; lane 2, MDA-MB-231; lane 3, T47 D; lane 4, MCF-7. Reprinted with permission from Anti-Cancer Research 1995; 15:295-304.

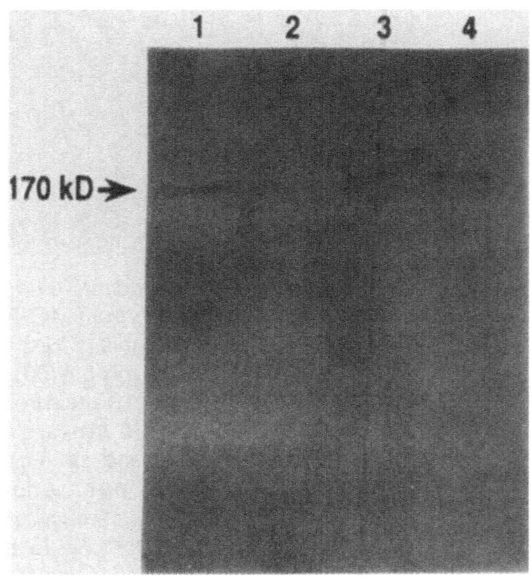

kD only) in cellular fractions from CHO cells also showed that the Topo II present in nuclear extract is representative of the Topo II present in the whole cell.[57] The amount of 170 kD enzyme was higher in MCF-7 and T47D cell lines, whereas MDA-MB-231 revealed no detectable Topo II in the whole cell lysates. It is noteworthy that both MCF-7 and T47D breast cancer cell lines are susceptible to pMC540 and merodantoin cytotoxicity. In addition, our results also show (Fig. 5.9) that m-AMSA, an inhibitor of Topo II, completely inhibited the decatenation activity in extracts from MDA-MB-231 at a concentration of 10 mM and in extracts from MCF-7 at a concentration of 40 mM.

These results clearly show that the formation of cleavable complex, and not pMC540, or merodantoin-induced inhibition of catalytic activity, plays a role in the lack of cytotoxicity. Thus, the reduced Topo II catalytic activity, reduced amounts of Topo II and the decreased formation of cleavable complex could account for the resistance of MDA-MB-231 cells to the cytotoxic action of pMC540 and merodantoin.

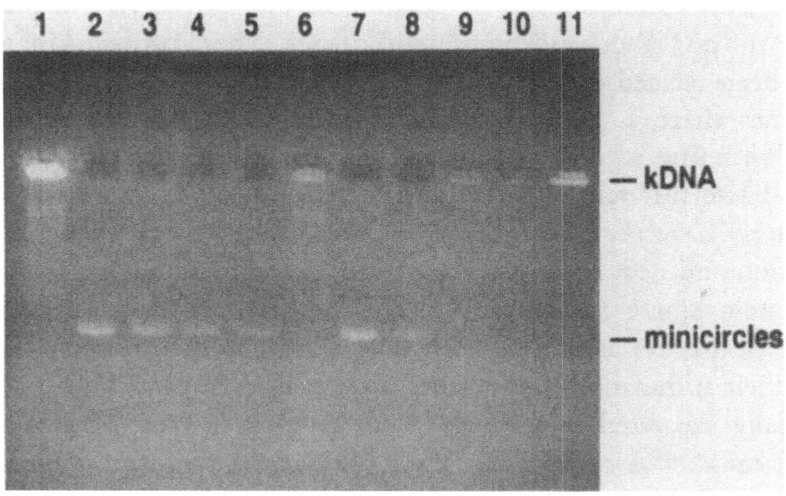

Fig. 5.9. Inhibition of the topoisomerase II activity in nuclear extract of MCF-7 and MDA-MB-231 by m-AMSA. Topoisomerase II activity was monitored by the decatenation assay as described earlier.[40] First various concentrations of m-AMSA were added to the reaction mixture (25 μl) containing 2.0 μg of kDNA and then 2.0 μg of nuclear extract protein from MCF-7 (lanes 2–6) or MDA-MB-231 (lanes 7–11) was added. After 30 min. at 37° C the reaction was terminated and analyzed. Lane 1, control, no drug, no extract protein; lane 2 and 7, control, no drug; lanes 3 and 8, 5 μM m-AMSA; lanes 4 and 9, 10 μM m-AMSA; lanes 5 and 10, 20 μM m-AMSA; lanes 6 and 11, 40 μM m-AMSA. Reprinted with permission from Anti-Cancer Research 1995; 15:295-304.

It is also important to note that in mammalian cells, there are two closely related isoforms of Topo II, called α and β, which are encoded on different chromosomes[58,59] and are apparently differentially regulated.[60] The α isoform is not a proteolysis product from the β isoform because peptide digestion products of these two isoforms are quite different and the antibodies raised against one form do not react with the other form. The heterogeneity of topoisomerases isoform function is incompletely understood. Our data presented above was obtained using purified 170 kD (α) human Topo II enzyme. The α isoform of this enzyme, but not the β isoform, is quantitatively associated with active cell growth.[61] It has been reported that isoform β represents 20-25% of total Topo II in proliferating cells.[60]

Therefore, from the data presented it is not possible to conclusively assign the dependence of pMC540 and merodantoin activity either to one or both isoforms of Topo II at this time. Similarly, it remains to be determined whether cyclic AMP-dependent protein kinase type I is involved in the observed Topo II dependent activity of pMC540 or merodantoin or not. In mammalian cells cAMP communicates by binding to one of the two distinct classes of cAMP-dependent protein kinases. These protein kinases have been termed type I and type II, respectively.[62] Both of these enzymes share a common catalytic subunit but differ in their cAMP-binding regulatory subunits. For protein kinase type I and type II two different R forms termed RIα, RIβ, RIIα and RIIβ respectively have been described.[62] A correlation between cell differentiation and neoplastic transformation with differential expression of protein kinase regulatory subunits has been reported.[63] Higher levels of RIα are associated with tumor cells or with normal cells after their stimulation with mitogenic stimuli, whereas RIIβ is preferentially expressed in normal tissues or quiescent or growth arrested cells.[63-66] A correlation between hypersensitivity of Topo II-targeting drugs and cyclic AMP-dependent protein kinase type I has been reported.[66] Further research is necessary to determine the role of cAMP-dependent protein kinases in the Topo II dependent activity of pMC540 and merodantoin. It would also be interesting to determine whether over-expression of RIα gene is associated with the malignant cell hypersensitivity to these Topo II dependent compounds.

APOPTOSIS

Soon after the discovery of the process of preactivation, concerted efforts were made to gather as much data as possible to document the effects of our lead compound pMC540 on cultured tumor cells. One set of such experiments involved the examination of the ultrastructure of untreated and pMC540 treated human lymphoma Daudi cells. Analysis of these electron microscopy data revealed evidence of apoptosis, such as chromatin condensation, blebbing of the plasma membrane and the nuclear envelope in these cells.[67,68] Apoptosis or physiological suicide has been recognized since the early days of embryology but was first emphasized by Glucksmann[69] and subsequently re-recognized in the 1960s. It is a process by which unwanted cells are removed from embryonic, developing or somatic tissue functions.[70-73] It was postulated that these cells contained a program or biological clock set for death well prior to the time the program was actually executed. A classic example of apoptotic death giving rise to the concept of the biological death-clock comes from the study of regulation of cell death of the posterior necrotic zone of chicken wings. These cells die in stage 24 of embryonic development. Until this time, it was impossible to distinguish them from their neighbors.[74] Another example of apoptotic death would be the loss of the tale of a tadpole as it matures into a frog. Yet another example comes from metamorphosing moths, where death of specific larvae or pupal neurones is known to occur in a specific sequence as each cell follows its own timing and sequence of death.[75-77]

Induction of this program or apoptosis appears to require a triggering event. In many cases it is a hormone or growth factor. For example, hormone-dependent apoptosis has been reported in the adrenal cortex following withdrawal of adrenocorticotropic hormone,[78, 79] in the prostate in the absence of testosterone,[80] in the endometrium[81] and in the breast epithelium.[82,83]

It has been reported that most anticancer drugs as well as irradiation and hormone therapy in current use induce apoptosis in tumor cells, although high doses may also cause cell death by other means.[84-86] An overview of apoptosis as a regulator of cell numbers in normal and neoplastic tissues and its significance in cancer and cancer therapy has been recently reported.[87-88] However the manner in which therapeutic agents induce apoptosis is not known. From the initial interaction of the apoptosis inducing agent with the target cell to the end point of cell death a multi-step process is involved. Some of the known events that occur in this process appear to include activation of endogenous calcium- and magnesium-dependent endonuclease that cleaves host chromatin into fragments. The occurrence of internucleosomal DNA fragmentation producing approximately 200 base pair fragments which appear as a ladder on DNA gels, remains the hallmark of apoptosis. However, despite this belief, new evidence continues to appear in the literature which suggests that this laddering effect indeed is not the case for all cells.[71, 89, 90] For example, other forms of DNA degradation not involving DNA strand breaks have been shown to occur in C3H/IOT$^{1/2}$ cell.[91] Generation of high molecular weight DNA fragments, detected only by pulse field electrophoresis, have been reported for glucocorticoids which induce apoptosis by a receptor mediated mechanism.[71, 92] According to these reports, high molecular weight DNA fragmentation may be a more universal marker for apoptosis than the so-called classical ladder formation. Indeed, our own experience with pMC540, merocil and merodantoin is in agreement with these findings because treatment of Daudi lymphoma cells with these agents caused an initial high molecular weight DNA fragmentation. Only prolonged incubation of these cells with pMC540, merocil or merodantoin led to the classical ladder formation. Nonetheless, other pathways, such as changes in the intracellular pH leading to the activation of deoxyribonucleases, have been reported.[93] It is now widely recognized that mere demonstration of anticancer drug X inducing apoptosis in cell type Y does not address the central issue of why these drugs cause cell death and why, sometimes, they do not. Towards this end, good studies are emerging and they have shown that protein p 26 encoded by the *bcl-2* gene inhibits apoptosis, a common mechanism of cell death which can be activated by multiple mechanisms including hormone and chemotherapy.[94, 95] More recently, studies by Jacobson et al[96] suggest that in many cells the molecular instruction for programmed cell death lie in the cytoplasm. In these studies cultured human fibroblast cells were treated with cytochalasin B to disrupt the cytoskeleton and later these cells were centrifuged until the nuclei popped out of the cell leaving behind an enucleated cytoplast. Treatment of these cytoplasts with staurosporine, a protein kinase inhibitor that induces cell death, caused morphological changes associated with programmed cell death. These studies were repeated in cytoplasts obtained from fibroblast cells expressing *bcl-2.* In these experiments morphological changes associated with programmed cell death were blocked by *bcl-2,* indicating that cells do not need a nucleus to undergo programmed cell death. Thus the nucleus may be just another target for destruction since proteins necessary to induce programmed cell death are already present in the cytoplasm.[96] It is, however, unlikely that programmed cell death in the absence of the nucleus is the final word for all types of cells. It may be that in certain types of cells such as embryonic cells where cell death does not have to be a rapid event, the proteins necessary for the induction of programmed cell death are synthesized after the signal is received. In this case, presence of the nucleus would be essential. More recent data regarding the involvement of other players such as p53 gene; bax, a 21 kD protein with homology to *bcl-2* gene; fas/APO-1, a member of the nerve growth factor/TNF-R superfamily; tumor necrosis factor; WAF1, a protein which functions to regulate the activity of cyclin dependent kinase (cdk2); interleukin-1β, and interleukin-1β-converting enzyme (ICE) to name a few, in the cascade of apoptosis are rapidly emerging.[97] Thus, our understanding of the complex mechanisms involved in the process of apoptosis is in a state of constant flux. As a result of this rapid expansion, the knowledge base is constantly changing. However, it is clear that multiple protein-protein interactions are involved in this important physiological process.

APOPTOSIS INDUCED BY pMC540, MEROCIL AND MERODANTOIN

In our previous studies we have shown that pMC540, merocil and merodantoin, are effective in causing a rapid (starting within 30 minutes of drug exposure) inhibition of macromolecular synthesis, indicating that they inhibit both mitotic and proliferative activities. The precipitous early decline in radioactive thymidine incorporation into cells treated with these agents indicates that these cells do not progress into the S phase of the cell cycle.[44, 68] These compounds were also found to be effective in inducing apoptosis in target cells tested.[44] For example, treatment of Daudi lymphoma cells with these agents for 30 minutes or 2 hours results in the formation of high molecular weight DNA cleavage. However, continued exposure of these cells for a period of 4 or 6 hours results in considerable DNA fragmentation as evidenced by the characteristic DNA laddering effect seen in agarose gels (Fig. 5.10). The high molecular weight DNA fragmentation observed at 30 minutes or 2 hours could be inhibited by a two hour pretreatment of Daudi cells with actinomycin D which inhibits transcription, as well as cycloheximide which inhibits translation of mRNA. These agents were ineffective in preventing DNA fragmentation after 4 hours of drug treatment, suggesting that steps in the process of cell death have progressed to a point of commitment.

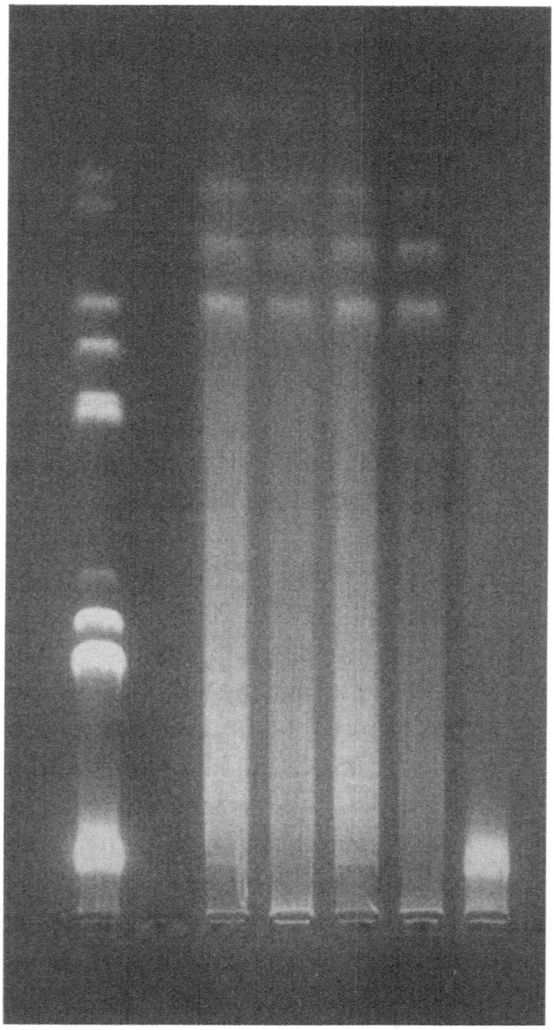

Fig. 5.10. Agarose gel electrophoretic pattern of DNA extracted from Daudi cells following exposure to pMC540, and merodantoin. Lane 1, untreated control; lanes 2 and 4, treated with pMC540; lanes 3 and 5, treated with merodantoin (4 hours and 6 hours, respectively). Lane 6, molecular weight markers (phage lambda-Hind III and ØX174 Hae III digest). Reprinted with permission from Anti-Cancer Drugs 1994; 5:557-566.

Many cytotoxic drugs that induce apoptosis also elevate the levels of intracellular calcium. It is generally believed, that early elevation of intracellular calcium provides a signal for the activation of endonucleases which finally cause DNA fragmentation. Therefore, we investigated the role of intracellular calcium in response to pMC540, merocil and merodantoin treatments. Only pMC540 treatment caused an elevation of intracellular calcium in Daudi cells and the effect occurred only after a 2 hour treatment with pMC540 (Fig. 5.11). These results suggest that: 1) involvement of intracellular calcium may be providing a signal to activate endonucleases since DNA fragmentation occurs at 4 or 6 hours and 2) since pMC540 contains meroxazole, merocil and merodantin, it is possible that the combined effect of more than one product may be responsible for the modulation of intracellular calcium. However, these and other possibilities remain to be explored.

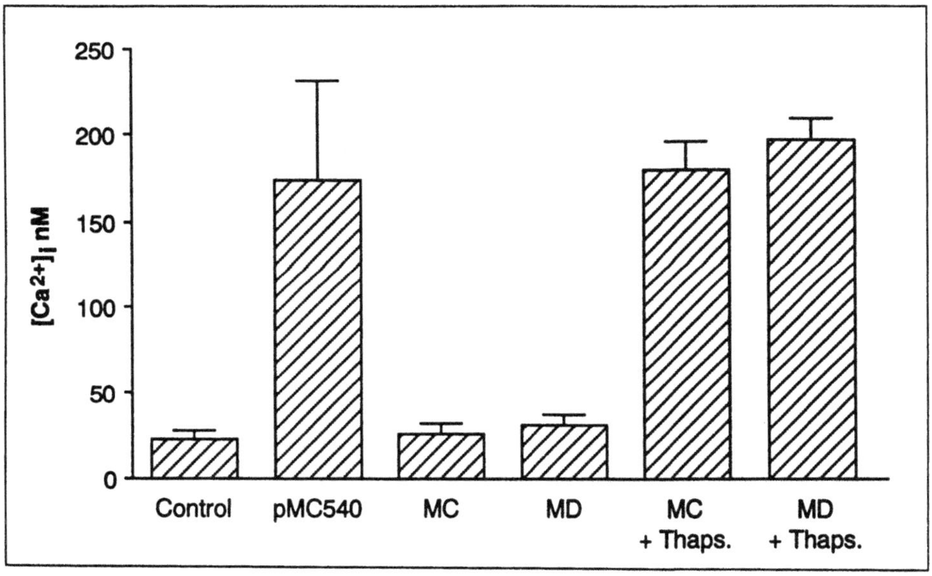

Fig. 5.11. Washed and Fura-2-AM-loaded Daudi cells (1 x 10^6 cells/ml) were treated with pMC540, merocil (MC), merodantoin (MD), MC plus thapsigargin (Thaps), or MD plus thapsigargin followed by washing and resuspension in Fura-2-AM buffer. Fluorescence of cellular suspension was measured alternatively at 340 nm_{ex}, 380 nm_{ex}, and 510 nm_{em}. Intracellular calcium concentration was calculated from the ratio of observed fluorescence intensities. Values are the mean ± SD of four separate experiments. Reprinted with permission from Anti-Cancer Drugs 1994; 5:557-566.

EFFECT OF pMC540 AND MERODANTOIN ON MITOCHONDRIAL MORPHOLOGY AND FUNCTION

To further enhance our understanding of the underlying mechanism of action, we chose to determine the effect of pMC540 and merodantoin on intact mitochondria. For this purpose, MCF-7 human breast cancer cells were used because of their anchorage dependent growth as well as their susceptibility to the cytotoxic action of these compounds. Rhodamine release from prestained cells has been shown to be caused by compounds that are respiratory poisons or ionophores.[98] Rhodamine 123 is a fluorescent cation that selectively localizes to mitochondria and its retention is dependent on the maintenance of the negative electrochemical gradient across the mitochondrial membrane. Thus, the effects of pMC540 and merodantoin on the intact mitochondria were further examined by monitoring the release of rhodamine 123 from preloaded MCF-7 cells in response to the drug treatments. Fluorescence microscopy of rhodamine-loaded control and treated cells revealed (Fig. 5.12A-B) that pMC540 treatment caused markedly diminished fluorescence emanating from drug treated cells as compared to the untreated controls.[99] These observations were further verified by spectrophotometric monitoring of the release of this dye in response to the pMC540 treatment. Results from this study clearly show that pMC540 induces a dose dependent release of rhodamine 123 from preloaded MCF-7 cells. As much as 70% of the dye was released from drug treated cells over a period of 7 hours (Fig. 5.13). This effect of pMC540 and merodantoin on mitochondria of intact cells was confirmed by studies of the electron microscopy, oxygen consumption, cellular ATP content and measurement of succinate dehydrogenase activity.

Electron microscopy of untreated and treated MCF-7 cells was compared. Results showed that in control cells euchromatin and

Fig. 5.12. (see opposite page) (A) Fluorescence micrograph of untreated (control) MCF-7 human breast cancer cells in culture stained with rhodamine 123. Bright fluorescence was predominantly distributed in the mitochondria of cells which fluoresce as small cytoplasmic bodies. (B) Fluorescence micrograph of pMC540 (210.5 μM) treated MCF-7 human breast cancer cells. Cells were stained with rhodamine 123 and examined following a 10, 20, 30, 60 and 120 minute treatment with pMC540. Photograph was taken after a 30 minute treatment showing less fluorescence of the majority of mitochondria as well as loss of nuclear detail. Similar results were obtained after treatment of MCF-7 cells with 103.3 μM merodantoin (photograph not shown). Reprinted with permission from Anti-Cancer Drugs 1995; 6:545-552.

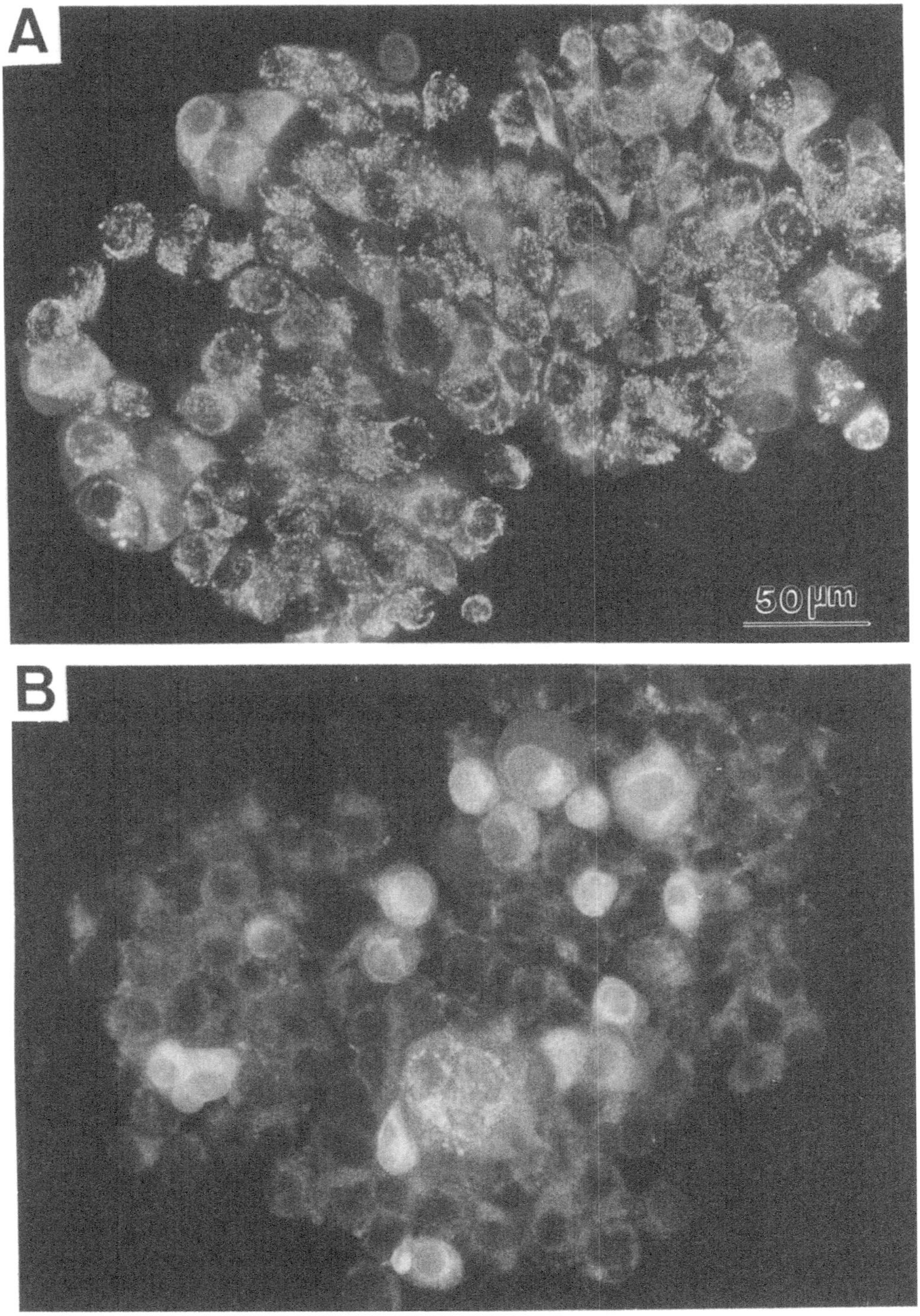
A
50 µm
B

prominent nucleolus in the nucleus and mitochondria with intact cristae were clearly visible in the cytoplasm of the cell (Fig. 5.14A). However, in pMC540 and merodantoin cells the mitochondria were swollen displaying various stages of damage. For example, in these cells: the matrix was less granular; cristae was discontinuous and it penetrated only a small portion of the interior of the mitochondrial membrane and the integrity of the outer mitochondrial membrane was lost resulting in the gradual collapse of the organelle and the eventual disruption of all membranous material (Fig. 5.14B). These structural changes in the mitochondria occurred following an incubation period as short as 60 minutes in the presence of pMC540 or merodantoin. This short period of

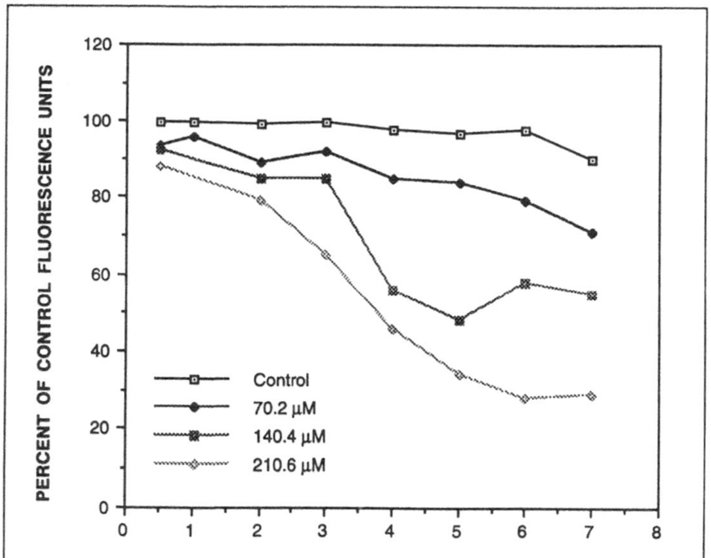

Fig. 5.13. Mitochondrial retention of rhodamine 123 in the absence and presence of different doses of pMC540. MCF-7 human breast cancer cells (5 x 10^5/ml) were plated in 12 well-culture dish, 1 ml per dish for 48 hours. The cells were loaded with 10 µg/ml rhodamine 123 for 10 min, and washed in PBS and then treated with 210.5 µM pMC540 and 103.3 µM merodantoin for 10, 20, 30 min, 1 hour and 2 hour. After the treatment, rhodamine retained in the cells was dissolved in 1 ml of 1% sodium dodecyl sulfate in distilled water for more than 1 hour. At time point of interest retained fluorescence was measured by a fluorescence spectrophotometer. Mean values of three separate experiments calculated as a percent of control fluorescent units are shown. Reprinted with permission from Anti-Cancer Drugs 1995; 6:545-552.

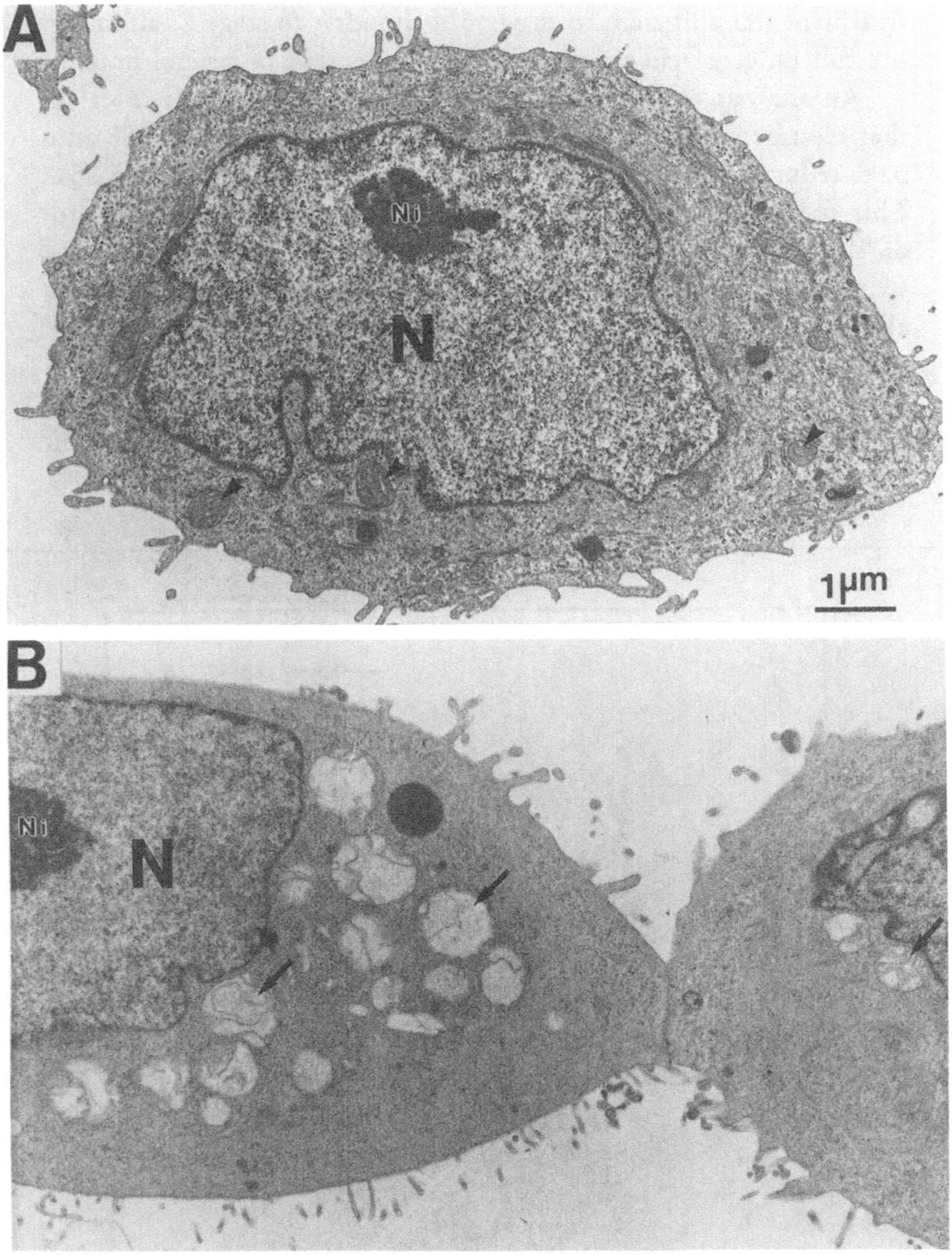

Fig. 5.14. (A) Electron micrograph of MCF-7 human breast cancer cells. A prominent nucleus (N) with euchromatin and a prominent nucleolus (Ni) is centered in cytoplasm containing small ovoid mitochondria (arrows) in condensed form occupied by cristae that traverse the mitochondrial matrix. (B) Electron micrograph of two MCF-7 human breast cancer cells following 8 hours incubation with 210.5 µM of pMC540. The nuclei (N) are more irregular in contour, the chromatin is more dispersed, and the nucleoli (Ni) are present. The cytoplasm contains swollen mitochondria showing disorientation or total loss in some cases of cristae (arrows). Reprinted with permission from Anti-Cancer Drugs 1995; 6:545-552.

treatment was sufficient to drive mitochondria to stage 2, although the full range of change occurred over a period of several hours.

An analysis of the cellular ATP levels in MCF-7 cells revealed that treatment with pMC540 and merodantoin caused a 49% and 32% reduction in cellular ATP levels within 15 minutes (Fig. 5.15). This reduction in ATP levels continued to decline over a period of 12 hours in a drug dose-dependent manner. Similarly, the activity of succinate dehydrogenase was reduced by 16% and 49% after a 30 minute and 2 hour treatment with pMC540 respectively (Fig. 5.16).

Next, oxygen consumption of drug treated and untreated cells was measured by using a Clarke oxygen electrode. Both total and

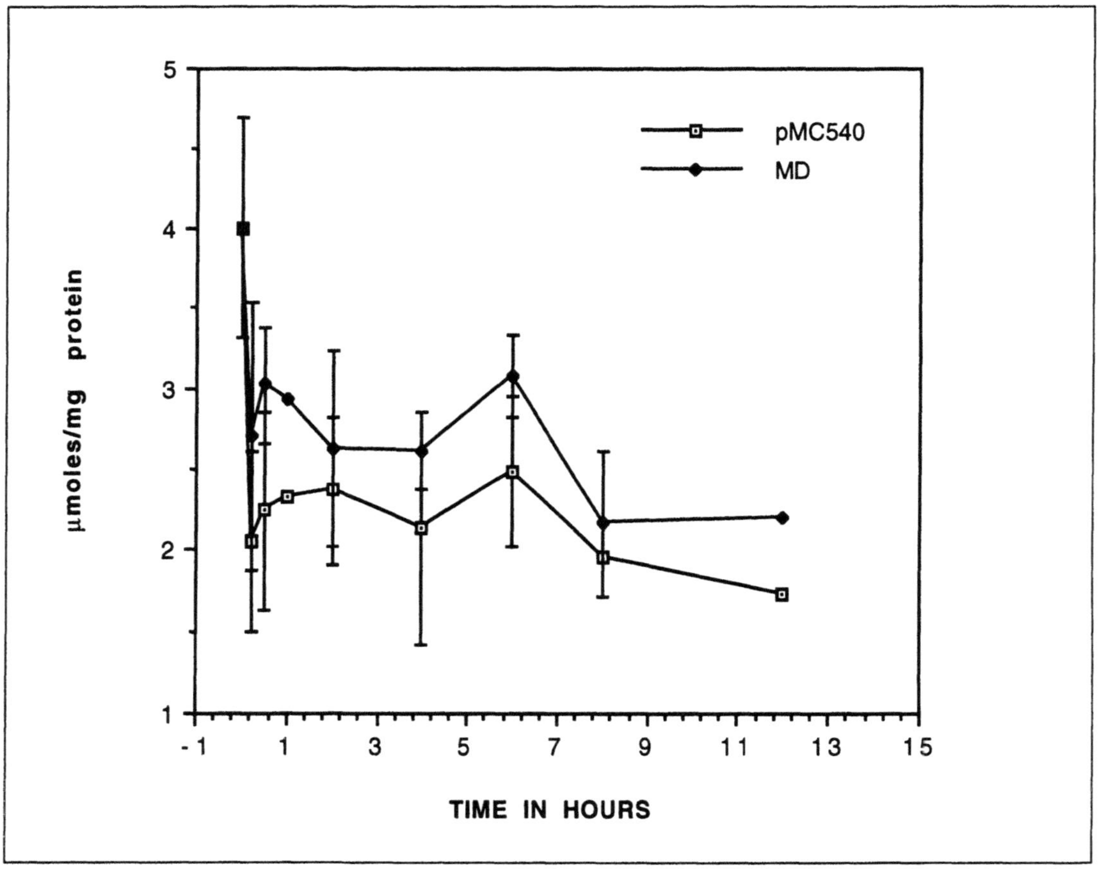

Fig. 5.15. Effect of pMC540 (210.5 µM) and merodantoin (103.3 µM) on the cellular ATP levels in MCF-7 human breast cancer cells treated for indicated periods of time. Mean ± S.D. of at least three separate experiments are shown. Reprinted with permission from Anti-Cancer Drugs 1995; 6:545-552.

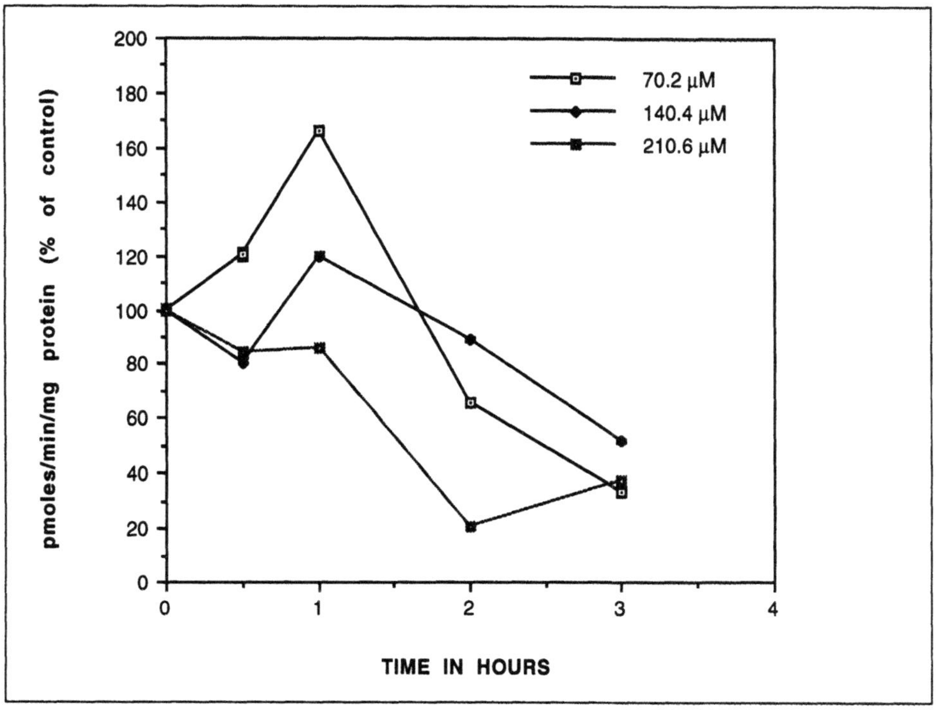

Fig. 5.16. Dose effect of pMC540 on in vitro activity of succinate dehydrogenase in MCF-7 human breast cancer cells. Data shown is percent of control values calculated from mean ± S.D. of three separate experiments each performed in triplicate. Reprinted with permission from Anti-Cancer Drugs 1995; 6:545-552.

cyanide resistant respiration were measured and mitochondrial respiration was calculated by subtracting the cyanide resistant respiration values from the total respiration values. Treatment of MCF-7 cells with pMC540 and merodantoin caused a marked and rapid reduction in mitochondrial respiration within the first 15 minutes. This initial drop was followed by a 4 hour recovery period followed by another decline in mitochondrial respiration which continued to drop over a period of 24 hours (Fig. 5.17). Taken together these data clearly demonstrate that mitochondria may be one of the key intracellular targets involved in the induction of cytotoxic effects mediated through disruption of energy balance by the action of pMC540 and merodantoin.

In conclusion, the data presented here demonstrate that novel chemotherapeutic agents used in this study mediate their cytotoxic effects via initial interaction with topoisomerase II eventually

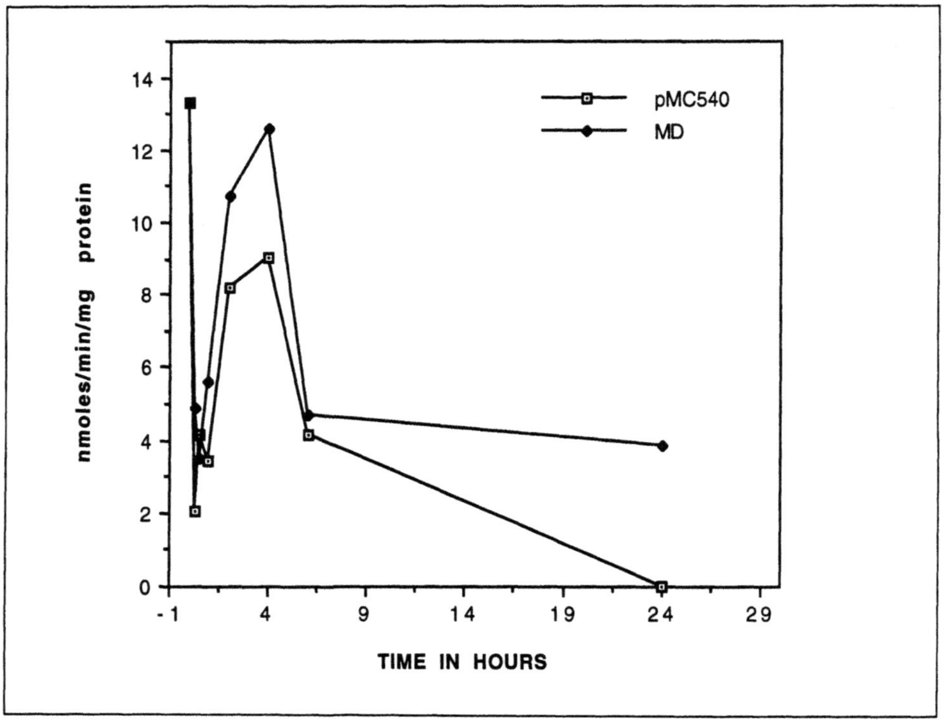

Fig. 5.17. Effect of pMC540 (210.5 μM) and merodantoin (103.3 μM) on oxygen consumption in MCF-7 human breast cancer cells. Three separate experiments were performed in triplicate to determine the total and cyanide resistant respiration. The values of total KCN resistant respiration were subtracted from the total cellular respiration values to obtain total mean values of mitochondrial oxygen consumption shown. Reprinted with permission from Anti-Cancer Drugs 1995; 6:545-552.

leading to apoptosis. Although, some involvement of reactive oxygen species in the observed biological activities of these compounds is likely, a conclusive case of their involvement based upon the data obtained thus far is not possible.

References

1. Halliwell B, Gutteridge JMC. Free Radicals in Biology and Medicine. Oxford: Clarendon, 1985.
2. McCord JM, Fridovich I. Superoxide dismutase. An enzymeic function for erythrocuprein (hemocuprein). J Biol Chem 1969; 244:6049-55.
3. Babior BM. Oxidants from phagocytes: agents of defense and destruction. Blood 1984; 64 959-66.
4. Comporti M. Lipid peroxidation and cellular damage in toxic liver injury. Lab Invest 1985; 53:599-623.

5. Gilbert DL, ed. Oxygen and Living Processes. An interdisciplinary approach. New York: Springer-Verlag, 1981.
6. Taeishi T, Yoshimine N, Kucuya F. Serum lipid peroxide assay by a new colorimetric method. Exp Gerontol 1987; 22:103-11.
7. Pervaiz S, Harriman A, Gulliya KS. Protein damage by photoproducts of merocyanine 540. Free Rad Biol & Med 1992; 12:389-96.
8. Davies KJA, Delsignore ME, Lin SW. Protein damage and degradation by oxygen radicals. J Biol Chem 1987; 262:9902-7.
9. Davies KJA and Delsignore ME. Protein damage and degradation by oxygen radicals. J Biol Chem 1987; 262:9908-13.
10. Davies KJA, Lin S, and Pacifici RE. Protein damage and degradation by oxygen radicals. J Biol Chem 1987; 262:9914-20.
11. Gross AJ, Sizer IW. The oxidation of tyramine, tyrosine, and related compounds by peroxidase. J Biol Chem 1959; 234:1611-14.
12. Prutz WA, Butler J, Land EJ. Phenol coupling initiated by one-electron oxidation of tyrosine units in peptides and histones. Int J Radiat Biol Relat Stud Phy Chem Med 1983; 44:183-96.
13. Bohlen P, Stein S, Dairman W, et al. Fluorometric assay of proteins in the nanogram range. Arch Biochem Biophys 1973; 155:213-20.
14. Thor H, Smith MT, Hartzel P et al. The metabolism of menadione (2-methyl-1,4-naphtholquinone by isolated hepatocytes. J Biol Chem 1982; 257:12419-25.
15. Doroshow JH. Role of hydrogen peroxide and hydroxide radical formation in the killing of Ehrlich tumor cells by anticancer quinones. Proc Natl Acad Sci USA, 1985; 83:4515–18.
16. Arslan P, Di Virgilio F, Beltrame M. Cytosolic Ca^{2+} homeostasis in Ehrlich and Yoshida carcinomas. J Biol Chem 1985; 260: 2719-27.
17. Mello Filho AC, Hoffmann ME, Meneghini R. Cell killing and DNA damage by hydrogen peroxide are mediated by intracellular iron. Biochem J 1984; 218:273-75.
18. Rosen H, Klebanoff SJ. Role of iron and ethylenediaminetetraacetic acid in the bactericidal activity of a superoxide anion-generating system. Arch Biochem Biophys 1981; 208:512-19.
19. Bates DA, Winterbourn CC. Deoxyribose breakdown by the adriamycin semiquinone and H_2O_2: evidence for hydroxyl radical participation. FEBS Lett 1982; 145:137-42.
20. Ward PA, Till GO, Kunkel R et al. Evidence for role of hydroxyl radical in complement and neutrophil-dependent tissue injury. J Clin Invest 1983; 72:789-801.
21. Rowe TC, Chen GC, Hsiang V et al. DNA damage by antitumor acridines mediated by mammalian DNA topoisomerase II. Cancer Res 1986; 46:2021-26.
22. Yang L, Rowe TC, Liu LF. Identification of topoisomerase II as the intracellular target of antitumor epipodophyllotoxins in simian virus 40 infected monkey cells. Cancer Res 1985; 45: 5872-76.

23. Hsiang YM, Lin ZF. Identification of mammalian DNA topoisomeras I as an intracellular target of the anticancer drug Camptothecin. Cancer Res 1988; 48:1722-26.
24. Wall ME, Wani MD, Cook CE et al. Plant antitumor agens. I. the isolation and structure of camptothecin, a novel leukemia and tumor inhibitor from *Camptotheca acuminata.* J Am Chem Soc 1966; 88:3888-90.
25. Perdue RE Jr, Smith RL, Wall ME et al. *Camptotheca acuminata* Decaisne (Nyssaceae). Source of campothecin. U S Dept \Agr, Agr Research Service 1970; Technical Bulletin No. 1415:1-26.
26. Heckendorf AH, Mattes KC, Hutchinson CR et al. Sterochemistry and conformation of biogenetic precursors of indole alkaloids. J Org Chem 1976; 41:2045-47.
27. Moertel CG, Schutt HJ, Reitmerer RJ et al. Phase II study of campthecin (NSC-100880) in the treatment of advanced gastrointestinal cancer. Cancer Chemother Rep Part I 1972; 56:95.
28. Gottleib JA, Luce JK. Treatment of malignant melanoma with camptothecin (NSC-100880). Cancer Chemother Rep 1972; 56:103.
29. Wani MC, Ronman PE, Lindley JT et al. Plant antitumor agents. 18. Synthesis and biological activity of camptothecin analogs. J Med Chem 1980; 23:554-60.
30. Andoh T, Ishii K, Suzuki Y et al. Characterization of mammalian mutant with camptothecin-resistant DNA topoisomerase I. Proc Natl Acad Sci USA 1987; 84:5565-69.
31. Gupta RS, Gupta R, Eng B et al. Camptothecin-resistant mutant of Chinese hamster ovary cells containing a resistant form of topoisomerase I. Cancer Res 1988; 48:6404-10.
32. Per SR, Mattern MR, Mirabelli CK et al. Characterization of a subline of P388 leukemia resistant to amsacrine: Evidence of altered topoisomerase II function. Mol Pharmacol 1987; 32:17-25.
33. Robson CN, Hoban PR, Harris AL et al. Cross-sensitivity to topoisomerase II inhibitors in cytotoxic drug-hypersensitive Chinese hamster ovary cell lines. Cancer Res 1987; 47:1560-65.
34. Wang JC. DNA topoisomerases. Annu Rev Biochem 1985; 54:665-97.
35. Vosberg HP. DNA topoisomerases: Enzymes that control DNA conformation. Curr Top Microbiol Immunol 1985; 114:19-102.
36. Osheroff N. Biochemical basis for the interaction of type I and type II topoisomerases with DNA. Pharmacol Ther 1989; 41:223-41.
37. D'Arpa P, Liu LF. Topoisomerase-targeting antitumor drugs. Biochim Biophys Acta 1989; 989:163-77.
38. Liu LF. DNA topoisomerase poisons as antitumor drugs. Annu Rev Biochem 1989; 58:351-57.
39. Rowe TC, Chen GL, Hsiang YH et al. DNA damage by antitumor acridines mediated by mammalian topoisomerase II. Cancer Res 1986; 46: 2021-26.

40. Osheroff N, Zechiedrich EL. Calcium-promoted DNA cleavage by eukaryotic topoisomerase II: Trapping the covalent enzyme-DNA complex in an active form. Biochemistry 1987; 26:4303-9.
41. Gibson BS, Ross WE. DNA topoisomerase II: a primer on the enzyme and its unique role as a multidrug target in cancer chemotherapy. Pharmacol Ther 1987; 32:89-106.
42. Kohn KW, Pommier Y, Kerriga D et al. Topoisomerase II as a target of anticancer drug action in mammalian cells. Natl Cancer Inst Monogr 1987; 4:61-71.
43. Zwelling LA. Topoisomerase II as a target of antileukemia drugs: a review of controversial areas. Hum Pathol 1989; 3:101-12.
44. Gulliya KS, Franck B, Schneider U et al. Topoisomerase II-dependent novel antitumor compounds Merocil and Merodantoin induce apoptosis in Daudi cells. Anticancer Drugs 1994; 5:557-66.
45. Sharma R, Arnold L, Gulliya KS. Correlation between DNA topoisomerase II and cytotoxicity in pMC540 and merodantoin sensitive and resistant human breast cancer cells. Anticancer Res 1995; 15:295-304.
46. Marsh W, Center MS. Adriamycin resistance in HL-60 cells and accompanying modification of a surface membrane protein contained in drug-sensitive cells. Cancer Res 1987; 47:5080-86.
47. Bhalla K, Hindenburg A, Taub RN et al. Isolation and characterization of an anthracycline-resistant human leukemia cell line. Cancer Res 1985; 45:3657-62.
48. Beck WT, Cirtain MC, Danks MK et al. Pharmacological molecular, and cytogenetic analysis of "atypical" multidrug resistant human leukemic cells. Cancer Res 1987; 47:5455-60.
49. Sinha BK, Haim N, Dusre L et al. DNA strand breaks produced by etaposide (VP-16, 213) in sensitive and resistant human breast tumor cells; Implication for the mechanism of action. Cancer Res 1988; 48:5096-5100.
50. Ferguson PJ, Fisher MH, Stephenson J et al. Combined modalities of resistance in etoposide-resistant human KB cell lines. Cancer Res 1988; 48:5956-64.
51. Marini JC, Miller KG, Englund PT. Decatenation of kinetoplast DNA by topoisomerase II. J Biol Chem 1980; 255:4976-79.
52. Miller KG, Liu LF, Englund PT. A homogenous type II DNA topoisomerase from HeLa cell nuclei. J Biol Chem 1981; 256:9334-39.
53. Liu LF, Miller KG. Eukaryotic DNA topoisomerases: two forms of type I DNA topoisomerases from HeLa cell nuclei. Proc Natl Acad Sci USA 1981; 78:3487-91.
54. Muller MT, Spitzner JR, Di Donato JA et al. Single-stranded DNA cleavage by eukaryotic topoisomerase II. Biochemistry 1988; 27:8369-79.

55. Spitzner JR, Chung IK, Muller MT. Eukaryotic topoisomerase II preferentially cleaves alternating purine-pyrimidine repeats. Nucleic Acids Res 1990; 18:1-11.
56. Foglesong PD, Reckord C. Improved electrophoretic separation of supercoiled and relaxed DNA in the presence of ethidium bromide. Biotechniques 1992; 13:402-4.
57. Sullivan DM, Latham MD, Ross WE. Proliferation dependent topoisomerase II content as a determinant of antineoplastic drug action in human, mouse, and Chinese hamster ovary cells. Cancer Res 1987; 47:3973-79.
58. Tsai-Pflugfelder M, Liu LF, Liu A et al. Cloning and sequencing of cDNA encoding human DNA topoisomerase II and localization of the gene to chromosome region 17q 21-22. Proc Natl Acad Sci USA 1988; 85:7177-81.
59. Jenkins JR, Ayton P, Jones T et al. Isolation of cDNA clones encoding the β isozyme of human DNA topoisomerase II and localization of the gene to chromosome 3p24. Nucl Acid Res 1992; 20:5587-92.
60. Woessner RD, Mattern MR. Proliferation and cell cycle dependent differences in expression of the 170 kilodalton and 180 kilodalton forms of topoisomerase II in NIH 3T3. Cell Growth & Differ 1991; 2:209-14.
61. Drake FH et al.. Biochemical and Pharmacological properties of p170 and p180 forms of Topoisomerase II. Biochemistry 1989; 18:8154-60.
62. Taylor SS, Buechler JA, Yonemoto W. cAMP-dependent protein kinase: framework for a diverse family of regulatory enzymes. Annu Rev Biochem 1990; 59:971-1005.
63. Cho-Chung YS. Role of cyclic AMP receptor proteins in growth differentiation and suppression of malignancy: new approaches to therapy. Cancer Res 1990; 50:7093-7100.
64. Tortora G, Yokozaki H, Pepe S et al. Differentiation of HL-60 leukemia by type I regulatory subunit antisense oligodeoxynucleotide of cAMP-dependent protein kinase. Proc Natl Acad Sci USA 1991; 88:2011-15.
65. Rohlff C, Clair T, Cho-Chung YS. 8-cl-cAMP induces down-regulation of the RIα subunit and up regulation of RIβ subunit of cAMP-dependent protein kinase leading to type II holoenzyme-dependent growth inhibition and differentiation of HL-60 leukemia cells. J Biol Chem 1993; 268:5774-82.
66. Tortora G, Pepe S, Cirafici AM et al. THS-regulated growth and cell cycle distribution of rat thyroid cells involve type I isozyme of cAMP-dependent protein kinase. Cell Growth & Differ 1993; 4:359-65.
67. Totora G, Ciardiello F, Damiano V et al. Cyclic AMP-dependent protein kinase type I in hypersensitivity of human breast cells to topoisomerase II inhibitors. Clin Cancer Res 1995; 1:49-56.

68. Gulliya KS, Pervaiz S, Dowben RM et al. Tumor cell specific dark cytotoxicity of preactivated merocyanine 540: implications for systemic therapy without light. Photochem Photobiol 1990; 52:831-38.
69. Glucksmann, A. Cell death in normal vertebrate ontogeny Biological Reviews 1951; 26:59-86.
70. Kerr JFR, Wyllie AH, Currie AR. Apoptosis: a biological phenomenon with wide-ranging implications in tissue kinetics. Br J Cancer 1972; 26:239-57.
71. Wyllie AH, Kerr JFR, Currie AR. Cell death: the significance of apoptosis. Int Rev Cytol 1980; 68:251-306.
72. Wyllie AH. Glucocorticoid-induced thymocyte apoptosis is associated with endogenous endonuclease activation. Nature (London) 1980; 284:555-56.
73. Kerr John FR, Winterford Clay M, Harmon Brian V. Its significance in cancer and cancer therapy. Cancer 1994; 73:2013-26.
74. Fallon JF, Saunders JW. In vitro analysis of the control of cell death in a zone of prospective necrosis from the chich wing bud. Developmental Biology 1968; 18:553-70.
75. Schwartz LM, Truman JW. Peptide and steroid regulation of muscle degeneration in an insect. Science 1982; 215:1420-21.
76. Truman JW. Programmed cell death in the nervous system of an adult insect. Journal of Comparative Neurology 1983; 216:445-52.
77. Truman JW. Schwartz LM. Insect systems for the study of programmed neuronal death. Neuroscience Commentaries 1982; 1:66-72.
78. Wyllie AH, Kerr JFR, Currie AR. Cell death in the normal neonatal rat adrenal cortex. J of Path 1973; 111:255-61.
79. Wyllie AH, Kerr JFR, MacAskill IAM, Currie AR. Adrenocortical cell deletion: The role of ACTH. J of Path 1973; 111:85-94.
80. Kerr JFR, Searle J. Deletion of cells by apoptosis during castration-induced involution of the rat prostate. Virchows Archiv (Cell Pathology) 1973; 13:87-102.
81. Sandow BA, West NB, Norman RL, Brenner RM. Hormonal control of apoptosis in hamster uterine lumina epithelium. American Journal of Anatomy 1979; 156:15-36.
82. Ferguson DJP, Anderson TJ. Morphological evaluation of cell turnover in relation to the menstrual cycle of the "resting" breast. British Journal of Cancer 1981; 44:177-81.
83. Ferguson DJP, Anderson TJ. Ultrastructural observations on cell death by apoptosis in the 'resting' human breast. Virchows Archiv (Pathology, Anatomy) 1981; 393:193-203.
84. Lennon SV, Martin SJ, Cotter TG. Induction of apoptosis (programmed cell death) in tumor cell lines by widely diverging stimuli. Biochem Soc Trans 1990; 18:343-51.
85. Kyprianou N, English HF, Davidson NE et al. Programmed cell death during regression of the MCF-7 human breast cancer following oestrogen ablation. Cancer Res 1991; 51:162-66.

86. Martikainen P, Kyprianou N, Tuker RW et al. Programmed cell death of nonproliferating androgen-independent prostatic cancer cells. Cancer Res 1991; 51:4693-4700.
87. Wyllie AH. Apoptosis and the regulation of cell numbers in normal and neoplastic tissues: an overview. Cancer Metastases Reviews 1992; 11:95-103.
88. Kerr FRJ, Winterford CM. Apoptosis; Its significance in cancer and cancer therapy. Cancer 1994; 73:2013-26.
89. Duke RC, Cohen JJ, Chervenak R. Differences in target cell DNA fragmentation induced by mouse cytotoxic T lymphocytes and natural killer cells. J Immunol 1986; 137:1442-47.
90. Ucker DS. Cytotoxic T-lymphocytes and glucocorticoids activate an endogenous suicide process in target cells. Nature (London) 1987; 327:62-64.
91. Tomei LD, Shapiro JP, Cope FO. Apoptosis in C3H/10T$^{1/2}$ mouse embryonic cells: evidence for internucleosomal DNA modification in the absence of double-strand cleavage. Proc Natl Acad Sci U S A 1993; 90:853-57.
92. Whitfield JF, Perris AD, Youdale Y. Destruction of the nuclear morphology of thymic lymphocytes by the corticosteroid cortisol. Exp Cell Res 1968; 52:349-62.
93. Eastman A. The pathway of apoptosis activated by anticancer agents. Proceedings of the American Association for Cancer Res 1992; 33:587-88.
94. Miyashita T, Reed JC. bcl-2 transfer increases relative resistance of S49.1 and WEHI7.2 lymphoid cells to cell death and DNA fragmentation induced by glucocorticoids and multiple chemotherapeutic drugs. Cancer Res 1992; 52:5407-541.
95. Hockenbery DM, Oltvai ZN, Yin X et al. Bcl-2 Functions in an antioxidant pathway to prevent apoptosis. Cell 1993; 75: 241-51.
96. Jacobsen MD, Burne JF, Raff MC. Programmed cell death and Bcl-2 protection in the absence of nucleus. EMBO J 1994; 13:1899-1910.
97. Steller H. Apoptosis- mechanisms and genes of cellular suicide. Science 1995; 267:1445-62.
98. Johnson LV, Walsh ML, Brokus BJ et al. Monitoring of relative mitochondrial membrane potential in living cells by fluorescence microscopy. J Cell Biol 1981; 88:526-35.
99. Gulliya KS, Sharma R, Liu HW et al. Relationship of mitochondrial function and cellular adenosine triphosphate levels to pMC540 and merodantoin cytotoxicity in MCF-7 human breast cancer cells. Anticancer Drugs 1995; 6:545-52.

CHAPTER 6

Modulation of Oncogenes with Preactivated Compounds

In previous chapters we have described the antitumor and antiviral properties of novel compounds discovered via the application of the process of preactivation. The studies of the mechanism of action of these compounds have also been summarized. In this concluding chapter, data from ongoing studies related to the effect of preactivated merocyanine 540 (pMC540) on the modulation of selected oncogenes will be discussed.

BACKGROUND

Research data from a large number of laboratories from all over the world have produced a general consensus that the development of cancer is a consequence of abnormal expression or function of specific cellular genes called oncogenes. Oncogenes were originally detected by their ability to induce neoplastic transformation. They have now been found to be mutant forms of normal cell genes called proto-oncogenes. Proto-oncogenes play a central role in regulatory systems governing the lives of normal cells. Therefore, the study of oncogenes and proto-oncogenes is important for the understanding of the molecular basis of cancer. Although cancer can be considered a collection of many diseases, there are common features in the development of different tumors that form the basis of our current understanding of carcinogenesis. Among the common features is the finding that most cancers arise from the transformation of a single cell. In human body, it is estimated that something on the order of 10^{16} cell divisions occur during a lifetime. Fundamental limitations on the accuracy of DNA replication and repair dictate that spontaneous mutations would occur at the rate of about 10^{-6} mutations per gene per cell division. Therefore, in a lifetime every single gene in the human body could be expected to mutate at about 10^{10} separate occasions. Among the resulting mutants or transformed cells, one could expect that normal regulatory controls and restrictions of cell divisions would be compromised yielding a transformed phenotype. The transformed phenotype is stably inherited at the time of cell division and continued proliferation produces a clonally derived population of cells. However, it is important to note that transformation of cell does not result from a single transforming event. As a matter of fact, the development of malignant phenotype is a complex multistage process which is clearly not understood. This view of multistage progressive alterations leading to malignant disease is supported by the observations that most cancers develop late in life and the incidence of the disease increases rapidly with age. For example, the death rate from colon carcinoma increases over one thousand fold between the ages of 30 and 80. This nonlinear response is inconsistent with the notion of a single event theory of transformation. The multistep nature of cancer development is also supported by the observations that precancerous or premalignant tissues are known to progress to a fully malignant stage.

Many of the different types of cancers studied have been demonstrated to correlate with genetic alterations which result in the activation of oncogene(s) or inactivation of a tumor suppressor gene(s).[1] However, other possibilities must also be kept in mind. A case in point is prostate cancer. It is well documented that prostate cancer occurs spontaneously only in man and dog. Prostate cancer never occurs in any other vertebrate animal species. The obvious question is why? Does this limitation apply only to prostate cancer or to other types of cancer as well? In 1995, there were approximately 38,000 deaths to prostatic cancer and 300,000 men underwent surgery for relief from benign prostatic hyperplasia. In contrast, there was not a single reported case of cancer of the seminal vesicles. This is remarkable, since like the prostate, the seminal vesicles are also members of the male sex accessory tissues, are responsive to androgens and share essentially the same blood supply and anatomical location in the body. Similarly, there has never been a documented case of cancer of the Cowper's gland located just below the prostate. If alteration in oncogenes or their function is the cause of cancer, the example of prostate cancer certainly forces one to consider other possibilities such as heritable epigenetic changes. In general, genetic alterations could occur at any stage of neoplastic transformation, resulting in heterogeneity of the tumor population. Thus, other factors in addition to the abnormal expression or function of oncogenes should be considered.

CHEMOTHERAPEUTIC DRUGS AND ONCOGENES

Many drugs are known to modulate the expression and function of oncogenes. For example, the treatment of Burkitt lymphoma Daudi cells with mechlorethamine causes suppression of *c-myc* expression, an early growth response gene, without affecting the *ras* expression.[2] Similarly, the expression of *c-myc* has been examined in response to a variety of antileukemic drugs.[3] Yet another example is the expression of *c-fos* which can be induced rapidly albeit transiently in a variety of normal cell types by a variety of agents such as growth factors, interleukins, tumor promoters such as phorbol esters, and neuroactive compounds.[4-8] Bifunctional agents such as 4-hydroxycyclophosphamide, L-phenylalanine mustard and mechlorethamine have also been reported to cause a profound suppression in the levels of *c-myc* transcripts but not the expression of N-*ras* or β-actin. In addition, differentiating agents such as dibutyryl cyclic AMP, dimethyl sulfoxide and 1,25-dihydroxyvitamin D3 are also known to reduce *c-myc* expression in certain tumor cell types prior to their terminal differentiation.[9-11]

In recent years, a number of investigations have shown that there is a strong association between expression of proto-oncogenes, cellular growth factors and the growth control of normal and neoplastic cells.[12] It also has been demonstrated that perturbations in normal cellular proto oncogenes can transform them into activated oncogenes. These changes could occur by a variety of mechanisms (e.g. amplification, translocation, point mutation) and typically result in aberrant gene expression or an altered gene product.[13-15]

Once activated, oncogenes appear to play a critical role in the tumorigenic phenotype.[16,17]

A paucity of data exists regarding the effects of clinically efficacious antitumor agents on oncogene expression. It is conceivable, however, that different antitumor agents may selectively inhibit the expression of specific oncogenes. For example, a preliminary report indicated that exposure to mechlorethamine suppressed *c-myc* expression but did not affect *ras* expression in the Burkitt lymphoma Daudi cell line.[18] Another report examined the effect of a variety of clinical antileukemic chemotherapeutic regimens on *c-myc* expression in patients with leukemia.[19] Because amplification of genes such as *myc, Her 2/neu* has been correlated with a poor prognosis[12-17], it could be inferred that overexpression of such genes contributes to tumor cell growth or survival. If overexpression of each of these genes contributes to tumorigenicity, strategies to decrease their expression may retard tumor growth.

EFFECT OF pMC540 ON *C-MYC* ONCOGENE IN LEUKEMIA

In view of this background information, involvement of *c-myc* in the pathogenesis of leukemia and lymphoma, and our findings of the marked sensitivity of human and mouse leukemia cells to the cytotoxic action of preactivated merocyanine 540 (pMC540), we elected to examine its effects on the expression of steady-state levels of *c-myc* oncogene mRNA and its protein products. In order to determine the appropriate drug dose for these studies, L1210 leukemia cells were first treated with varying doses of pMC540 for different periods of time. After the indicated duration, control and pMC540 treated L1210 cells were plated (in triplicates) in a clonogenic assay. Colonies consisting of 50 or more cells were counted on day 7. Analysis of the data obtained revealed that pMC540 at doses of 70.2 μM, 140.4 μM and 210.6 μM resulted in a significant ($p < 0.001$) inhibition of clonogenic growth of L1210 cells requiring 30 minutes to 16 hours of drug exposure (Fig. 6.1). The degree of growth inhibition was clearly drug dose and time dependent. Thus, these three drug doses producing varying degrees of cell kill were chosen for subsequent studies of *c-myc* regulation in response to pMC540 treatment.

DOWN REGULATION OF *C-MYC* BY pMC540

Next, the determination of *c-myc* transcripts in pMC540-treated and control cells was performed by Northern blot analysis. A total of 20 μg denatured RNA per well from control and drug-treated cells was analyzed on 1.2% formaldehyde/agarose gels and then transferred to a nitrocellulose paper. A ^{32}P-labeled *c-myc* probe (2.3-Kb, 3rd exon) with a specific activity of 1-2 x 10^8 cpm/μg was prepared by nick translation. Nitrocellulose filters with bound RNA were then boiled for 5 minutes in 20 mM Tris, pH 7.6, and pre-hybridized at 42°C for 12 hours in a solution of 50% deionized formamide, 5x standard saline citrate (SSC; x SSC-0.15 M NaCl/ 0.015 M trisodium citrate), 1% sodium dodecyl sulfate (SDS), 5x Denhardt's solution (50x = 1% Ficoll, 1% polyvinylpyrrolidone,

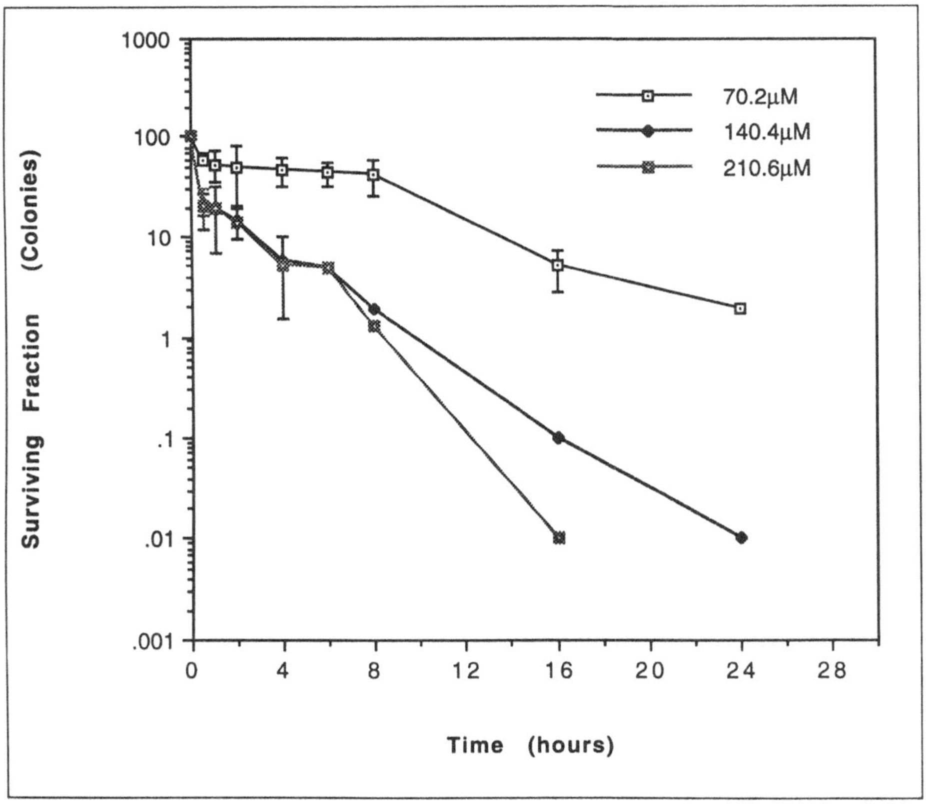

Fig. 6.1. Effect of pMC540 treatment on clonogenic growth of L1210 cells. L1210 cells (1 x 10^5 cells/ml) were treated with different doses of pMC540. After the indicated period of time, cells were washed and plated for colony formation assay. Results are mean ± S.E. of three separate experiments.

1% bovine serum albumin (BSA)), and 150 μg/ml denatured, sonicated salmon sperm DNA. For hybridization, the prehybridization solution plus probe at 42°C were used for 24 to 36 hours. Filters were then washed 4 times at room temperature for 5 minutes each in 2x SSC, 0.1% SDS, then twice at 55°C for 15 minutes each in 0.1x SSC, 0.1% SDS, and then twice at room temperature for 5 min each in 0.1x SSC. Filters were dried with a heat lamp, wrapped in plastic wrap, and autoradiographed using Kodak XAR-5 film and Lightning-Plus intensifying screens at –70°C. Signal intensity was measured by using a Shimadzu densitometer.

Northern blot analysis performed in this manner clearly shows (Fig. 6.2a) that the treatment of cells with 70.2 μM pMC540 produced a detectable reduction in *c-myc* transcripts after 4 hours of drug exposure. At higher concentrations of pMC540 (140.4 and 210.6 μM), a reduction of 1.8- and 5-fold, respectively, in *c-myc* transcripts was observed requiring only 1 hour of treatment. Next, we considered the possibility that the observed reduction in *c-myc* expression could be due to pMC540 induced cell death. However, this possibility was ruled out because identical amounts of mRNA were loaded onto the gels, and there was no correlation between the cell death (a 1 hour of pMC540 treatment at doses of 140.4 and 210.6 μM, produced a cell kill of 24% and 28% respectively) and the amount of reduction in *c-myc* transcripts. However, it is noteworthy that these reductions in *c-myc* transcripts were not detectable after 8 or 12 hours of drug treatment, suggesting a nearly complete shut down of transcription. In order to substantiate these findings, L1210 cells were treated with pMC540 for 6 hours and then layered on top of Ficoll-Hypaque density gradient. After centrifugation, living cells were collected and maintained in culture for 16 passages of cell growth in the absence of pMC540. Northern blot analysis performed at cell passage numbers 5, 7, 10, 13 and 15 revealed that *c-myc* transcripts could not be detected. However, *c-myc* transcripts were detectable at cell passage number 16, but the level of this expression was lower than the control levels of *c-myc* mRNA. These data suggest that a brief treatment of leukemia cells with pMC540 can cause a prolonged down regulation of *c-myc* transcription which was reversible under the conditions employed. Further confirmation of these findings by nuclear run-off assay remains to be done.

Control experiments were also done by using native (unactivated) merocyanine 540 (MC540). In these experiments, treatment of L1210 cells with unactivated MC540 (210.6 μM) did not cause observable reduction in the expression of *c-myc* up to 8 hours. However, after 24 hours of treatment a 1.6 fold reduction was observed. These very low levels of reduction in *c-myc* expression were probably due to non-specific activation of the compound occurring during various manipulations in room light.

Next, the effect of pMC540 on the expression of the constitutively expressed "housekeeping gene" β-actin was determined. Treatment of leukemic cells with pMC540 (70.2 μM and 140.4 μM) produced very little effect for up to 8 hours on β-actin (Fig. 6.2a). At higher concentrations (210.6 μM), the β–actin gene was affected

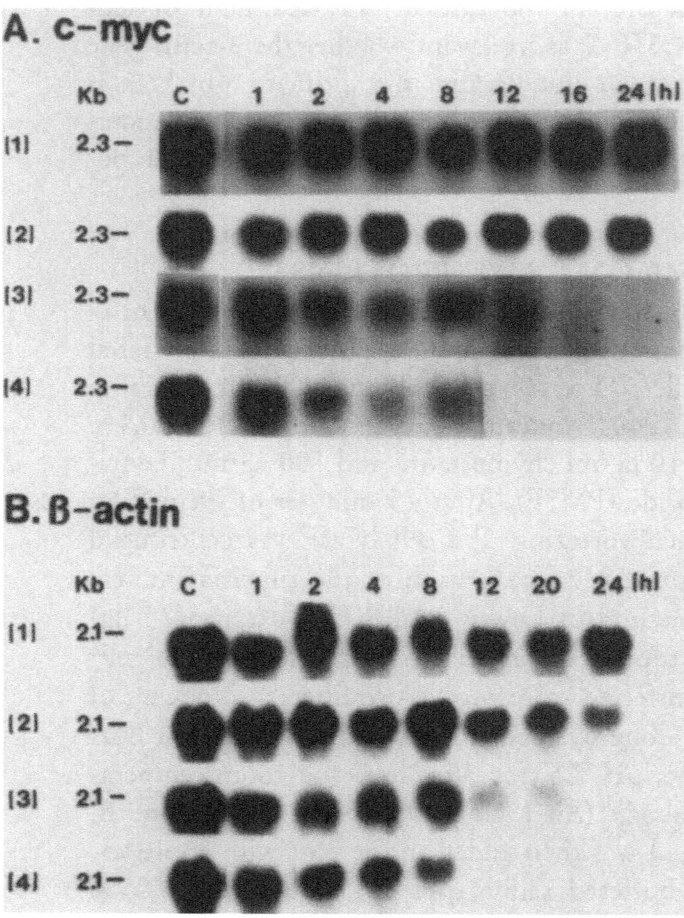

Fig. 6.2. Analysis of (a) c-myc and (b) β-actin mRNA expression in L1210 cells after MC540 and pMC540 treatment at the indicated periods of time. Each slot contains 20 μg of total cellular RNA. The same blot was probed for c-myc and β-actin. Lane 1, 210.6 μM MC540; lanes 2–4, 70.2, 140.4, and 210.6 μM pMC540.

after 1 hour of treatment (Fig. 6.2b). These results suggest that chromatin is affected by the action of pMC540 and β-actin is also affected. The specificity issue needs further elaboration here. Is the specificity of a drug, in terms of which genes are affected by it, important? The answer depends on the intended use of the drug. If one wants to selectively modulate or regulate a given oncogene in certain cells, then it is highly desirable that the effect of the drug is limited not only to the intended cells, but also to a specific gene within the cell. However, the main goal of any cancer therapy is to destroy the tumor cells and spare the host, i.e. normal cells and tissues. Thus, sparing of normal cells and tissues is of paramount importance in cancer therapy and one of the key points addressed in chapter 1. For pMC540 we have already demonstrated that it is very effective in killing certain types of malignancies and viral infections while very sparing of normal cells and tissues.[20-24] Therefore, in the case of the treatment of leukemia cells with pMC540, it is irrelevant whether the β-actin gene is affected by pMC540 or not because the ultimate aim here is the destruction of leukemic cells and enhancement of our understanding of the underlying molecular mechanism(s) for further potential exploitation.

EFFECT OF pMC540 ON C-MYC PROTEINS

Next the effects of pMC540 treatment on the expression of c-myc proteins were examined. Total protein extracts were prepared by lysing the cell pellets (5 x 10^7 cells/ml) in 2x PBS containing 1% Nonidet P40 (NP40), sodium deoxycholate (DOC), 0.1% SDS, 1 mM EDTA, 10 μg/ml chymostatin, and 100 μg/ml phenylmethylsulphonyl fluoride (PMSF). After 15 minutes of incubation at 4°C with occasional vortexing, the cell lysate was centrifuged (10,000 rpm). The protein concentration of the supernatant was determined by the method of Lowry et al.[25] Cell extract (25 μg) was resolved by electrophoresis on 12% SDS-polyacrylamide gel[26] and subsequently transferred to nitrocellulose filters.[27] Blocking of nonspecific sites was done by incubating the filters with 1% BSA in Tris-buffered saline, pH 7.5, for 30 minutes at room temperature. Anti–*c-myc* antibody (Ab-1 clone 9E10 and Ab-2 clone 8, Oncogene Science Inc.) was then added to the blot with appropriate dilution in Tris-buffered saline, pH 7.5, containing 0.05% Tween 20 (TBST). After 30 minutes of incubation at 25°C, the unbound antibody was removed by washing 3 times for 5 minutes each in TBST. Membranes were then transferred to TBST containing the 1:5000 dilution of mouse anti-IgG alkaline phosphatase conjugate as recommended by Promega's ProtoBlot II AP system with stabilized substrate for 30 minutes with gentle agitation. After 1 hour incubation with the second antibody, the membranes were washed as described above. The color development was initiated by incubating the membranes in Western blue stabilized substrate for alkaline phosphatase until the band of interest reached the desired intensity. Reactive areas turned purple, usually within 3–5 hours. Color development was terminated by washing the membranes in deionized water for several minutes, changing the water 2 to 3 times.

Results from these experiments show (Fig. 6.3a) that in cells treated with 70.2 μM pMC540, both 67-kD and 64-kD proteins are consistently present until 20 hours after the treatment. However, in cells treated with a dose of 140.4 μM (Fig. 6.3a), results suggest that the rate of 67 kD protein expression was significantly diminished at 8 hours and was barely detectable at 16 and 20 hours. Similar results were obtained in cells treated with 210.6 μM pMC540. Taken together these data suggest that the down-regulation of *c-myc* was followed (within a few hours) by a reduction in *c-myc* product. Because of the similarities in the kinetics of down-regulation of *c-myc* and 67 kD protein product, it appears that 67 kD protein may be involved in the translation of *c-myc* mRNA in L1210 cells. Figure 6.3a also shows the presence of c-myc proteins (67 kD and 64 kD) in the total cell protein. However, in pMC540-treated cells, 67 kD protein is reduced significantly, but 64 kD protein is not.

It is well established that c-myc proteins are predominantly localized in the nucleus of the cell. To determine whether pMC540 treatment affects the c-myc proteins in the cell nucleus or the cytoplasm, experiments were done to detect these proteins in subcellular fractions. For this purpose, subcellular fractionation of drug-treated and control cells (2 x 10^7), washed extensively in PBS, was carried out by a method described by Kaufmann et al.[28] Briefly, washed cells were pelleted and resuspended in STM (0.25 M sucrose, 50 mM Tris (pH 7.6), 5 mM $MgCl_2$) buffer containing 0.5% Trasylol-1 mM PMSF and 10 mM iodoacetamide. The cells were lysed immediately by 20–25 strokes in a glass Dounce

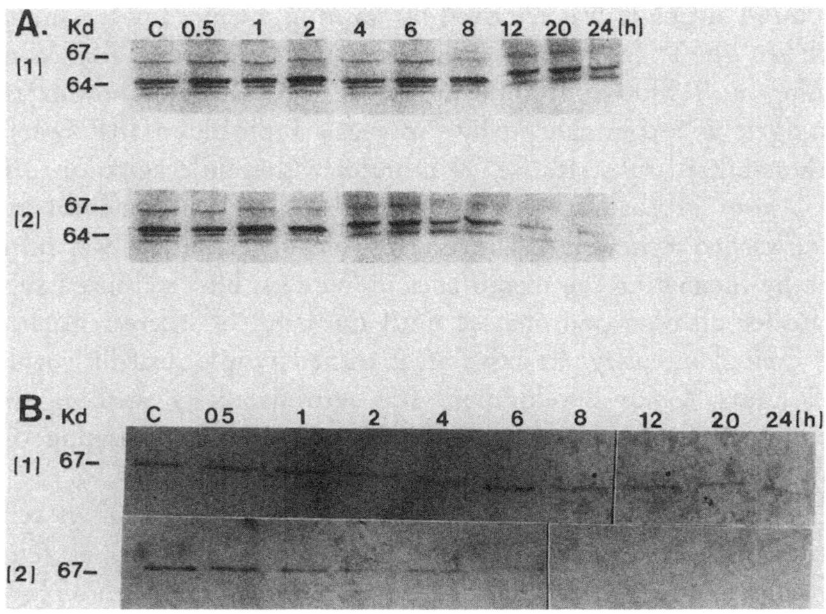

Fig. 6.3. Expression of c-myc protein in L1210 cells treated with pMC540 at the indicated periods of time. 25 µg of protein was electrophoresed. (A) Total cellular and (B) nuclear fraction protein from cells treated with 70.2 µM pMC540 (lane 1) and 210.6 µM pMC540 (lane 2).

homogenizer and centrifuged at low speed to pellet the nuclei. The supernatant represented the cytoplasmic fraction. Nuclei were washed 3 times in STM buffer and centrifuged through a 1 M sucrose cushion. The nuclear pellet then was resuspended in STM buffer containing 0.5% NP40 and 0.1% DOC and incubated for 15 minutes, then the nuclei were centrifuged at low speed. The resultant supernatant represented the nucleoplasmic fraction. The nuclei then were washed once in STM buffer containing 0.5% NP40 and 0.1% DOC. The final pellet represented the detergent-washed nuclei fraction. All three fractions (cytoplasm, nucleoplasm and nuclei) were adjusted to 0.5% NP40, 0.1% DOC and 0.5% SDS in STM buffer, sonicated briefly, freeze-thawed once and centrifuged at 10,000 x g for 10 minutes to pellet debris. After determination of the protein concentrations, the samples were subjected to SDS-polyacrylamide gel electrophoresis and Western blotting as described above. Results show (Fig. 6.3b) that 90% of the 67 kD protein associated with the nuclear fraction is affected by pMC540. The 64 kD protein was undetectable in the nuclear fraction. The 67 kD protein was not detectable in the nucleoplasm and cytosol fractions. To control for nonspecific association of 67 kD c-myc protein with the nuclear fraction, the subcellular fractionation was performed in a number of different ways, including detergent lysis or the use of spermine and spermidine to stabilize the cell nuclei.[29] Under all conditions employed, only 67 kD protein could be fractionated with the nuclei. These data suggest that 67 kD protein is more likely to be involved in the translation of *c-myc* mRNA in L1210 cells.

TUMORIGENESIS OF pMC540 TREATED BUT LIVING L1210 LEUKEMIA CELLS

The next set of experiments were performed to determine whether the pretreatment of L1210 cells with pMC540 prevents tumor growth in vivo. For this purpose, L1210 cells were first treated with 210.6 μM of pMC540 for 6 hours at 37°C. Under these conditions, 52% of the leukemic cells survived the treatment, as determined by the trypan blue exclusion method. After the incubation period, 1×10^5 treated and untreated living cells were injected into 2 month-old DBA/2 mice intraperitoneally, in groups consisting of 10 animals each. The animals were observed for a period of 3 months, and their survival times were recorded. The median survival time (when total number of animals [N] is even) was computed by using the formula: survival time (days) = $(X + Y)/2$, where X is the earliest day when the number of survivors is $\leq N/2$, and Y is the earliest day when the number of survivors is $\leq (N/2) - 1$. If N is odd, the median survival time is X.

Under the conditions employed, the median survival of control animals was 9 days, whereas the median survival of 54.5 days in the treated group was significantly ($p < 0.001$) enhanced (Fig. 6.4). At the end of the experiment (day 90), the L1210 cells retrieved from the ascites of the surviving animals (treated group) proliferated easily in in vitro cultures. These results suggest that the inhibition of the in vivo leukemia cell proliferation induced by pMC540 may be closely linked to the observed increased survival of animals receiving pMC540-treated leukemia cells. The down regulation of *c-myc* may also be an important factor in this scenario. Down-regulation of *c-myc* transcripts by a number of compounds, including alkylating agents (such as mechlorethamine, L-phenylalanine mustard and 4-hydroxycyclophosphamide) and differentiating agents (such as dibutyryl cyclic 3', 5'-AMP, dimethyl sulfoxide, 1,25-dihydroxyvitamin D) have been reported.[30] Similarly, it has been shown that interferon-alpha by itself and interferon-gamma in combination with tumor necrosis factor alpha can arrest tumor cell growth, which corresponds to the suppression of *c-myc* transcripts. Thus, down-regulation of *c-myc* expression induced by pMC540 treatment may be indicative of a loss of cell proliferation or a precursor event to cell killing, as in the case of nitrogen mustard.

The data presented here lend further support to the hypothesis that enhanced expression of *c-myc* confers upon tumor cells a higher malignant phenotype and may be one of the players in contributing to tumor progression. These results demonstrate that pMC540-mediated (in vitro) reduction of *c-myc* expression in L1210 cells results in a significantly reduced tumorigenicity in vivo.

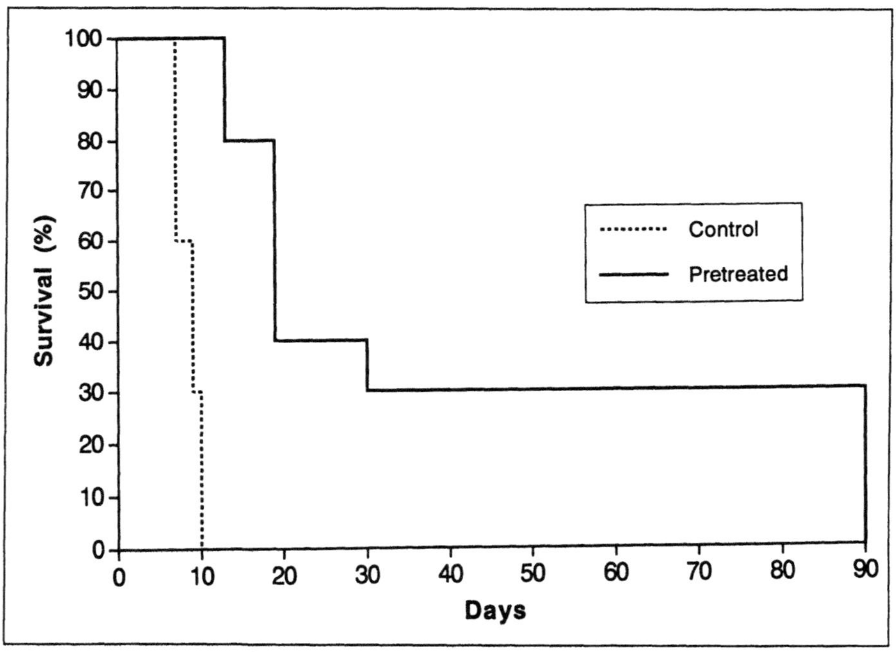

Fig. 6.4. The survival time of L1210-bearing mice after the pretreatment of implanted cells with pMC540. On day 0, 10^5 L1210 cells treated with pMC540 (210.6 µM) for 6 hours or untreated cells were injected intraperitoneally. Survival times for each group consisting of 10 animals each were recorded. The total observation period for survival time was 90 days.

STIMULATION OF TOPOISOMERASE II-INDUCED CLEAVAGE SITES IN *C-MYC* ONCOGENE BY pMC540

In previous studies (chapter 5) we have demonstrated that pMC540 mediated cytotoxicity involves an initial interaction with Topo II.[31,32] The Topo II enzyme is known to alter the DNA conformation by temporarily breaking and rejoining both DNA strands. We have shown that pMC540 traps Topo II in an intermediary complex with DNA, preventing the final rejoining step of this reaction. Single and double strand breaks were then visualized by analyzing the SDS-treated complex thus formed. These findings were consistent with the behavior of several other drugs such as 4' -(acridinylamino) methanesulfon-m-anisidide (m-AMSA), VM26, an acridine, and epipodophyllotoxin derivative, also known to interfere with mammalian Topo II, a predominant cause of their cytotoxic action.[33] Thus, in agreement with these reports, we summarized that pMC540-induced formation of Topo II-DNA complexes could be one of the major causes of its cytotoxic action.

In view of the findings that pMC540 interacts with Topo II and also down-regulates the expression of c-myc oncogene, the possibility that damage within select genomic regions may contribute to the antiproliferative activity of pMC540 was considered. This hypothesis was investigated by analyzing the differential damage in regions surrounding the *c-myc* locus in L1210 leukemia cells for the determination of DNA cleavage sites. In these experiments L1210 cells were treated with 70.2 μM and 140.4 μM pMC540 for a period of 8 hours and 12 hours. After this treatment DNA preparations from drug-treated and control cells were digested to completion with restriction enzyme (Hind III) and analyzed by Southern blot hybridization using the third exon of *c-myc* probe. Results of this analysis show (Figure 6.5A, lane 1) the banding patterns of DNA from untreated control cells. The banding patterns of pMC540-treated cells are shown in lanes 3-6. From these patterns it is clear that several hybridization bands of smaller size are visible in pMC540-treated DNA which could be related to the in situ *c-myc* gene cleavage products. It is noteworthy that in cells treated with unactivated merocyanine 540, cleavage bands were not observed (lane 2). In previous studies we have demonstrated that only pMC540 and not the native MC540, produces dose dependent dark cytotoxicity in certain types of tumor cells and this action involves an interaction with Topo II.[31,32] In order to determine whether the observed double stranded breaks in the c-myc oncogene were caused by pMC540-induced stimulation of Topo II, ethidium bromide, a known inhibitor of the formation of Topo II-DNA complex, was used.[34] Results from these experiments show that cells pretreated with 50 μM ethidium bromide for 30 minutes followed by a 3 hour treatment of these cells with 70.2 μM and 140.4 μM pMC540 failed to induce DNA cleavage (Figure 6.5A, lanes 8-9). Ethidium bromide in itself did not induce formation of cleavage bands (lane 7). Thus the observed cleavage of *c-myc* is dependent on pMC540-induced stimulation of Topo II. These cleavage sites generated by pMC540 treatment were mapped in the c-myc locus and the sites of preferential cleavage were located in the 5' part of the *c-myc* locus (arrow 5) and in the introns (arrows 1-4).

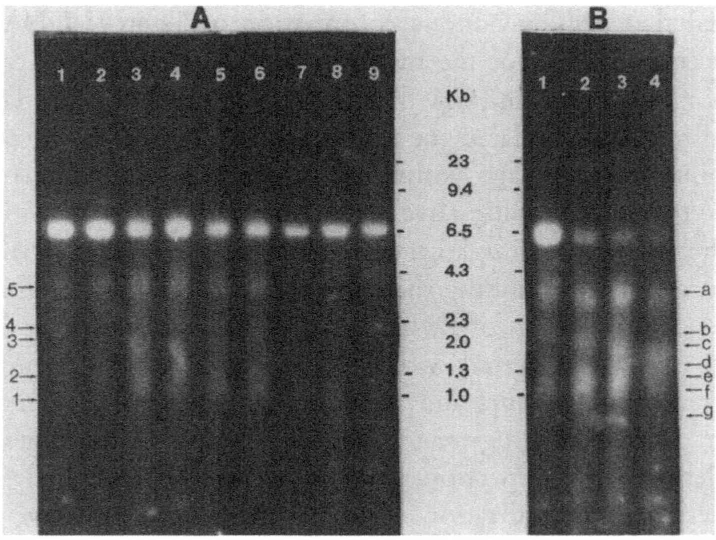

Fig. 6.5A. Cleavage sites induced in vivo by antitumor drug in the amplified c-myc gene of L1210 cells. DNA preparations (10 μg) from drug treated L1210 cells were digested with Hind III and analyzed by Southern blot hybridization using a 32p-labeled c-myc probe (third exon). 1:Untreated cells. 2: Treated with MC540 (100 μM). 3-4: pMC540 treated (70.2 μM 8 and 12h). 5-6: pMC540 treated (140.4 μM 8 and 12 h). 7: EthBr (50 μM). 8: EthBr (50 μM) + pMC540 (70.2 μM). 9: EthBr (50 μM) + pMC540 (140.4 μM); Fig. 6.5B. DNAse I hypersensitive sites determined in the amplified c-myc gene of L1210 isolated nuclei. DNA preparations (10 μg) were digested with Hind III and analyzed by Southern blot hybridization using c-myc (third exon). 1: Control nuclei. 2-4: Nuclei treated for 5 min at 37°C with 0.5. 1 and 2 μg/ml of DNAse I. The blots were exposed to Kodak XARS film to 3 days. DNA length fragments are given in kilobase pair (Kb). Reprinted with permission from Anti-Cancer Drugs 1996; in press.

For other Topo II-dependent drugs such as mAMSA, and VM-26 it has been shown that cleavable complex induced by these drugs preferentially occurs at the 5' noncoding end of the *c-myc* gene close to DNAase I hypersensitive cleavage sites.[35, 36] Therefore, an analysis of DNAase hypersensitive sites in the *c-myc* gene of L1210 cell isolated nuclei was performed according to previously described methods.[36] Results from these experiments revealed that pMC540-stimulated Topo II cleavage sites and DNAase I hypersensitive sites clearly appeared to map within the region of *c-myc*'s 5' end (Figure 6.5B). However, the two DNAase I hypersensitive sites (arrow c and d) have no Topo II cleavage site equivalents. In addition, experiments of the sensitivity of DNAse I made on the *c-myc* chromatin of quiescent cells (obtained under the conditions of serum deprivation) and growing L1210 cells yielded identical patterns of hypersensitive sites indicating that in the presence of pMC540 only a fraction of Topo II is capable of reacting with the *c-myc* chromatin, independently of the variation of Topo II activity. Another explanation of the observed in situ *c-myc* gene cleavage could be the dependence of the cleavage activity on the chromatin accessibility to nuclear proteins associated with the transcriptional activity of the gene. If true, this would also explain the relationship between the *c-myc* transcription and cleavage activity induced by pMC540. It is quite interesting that in further analysis of pMC540-treated L1210 cells, cleavage of other genes such as *c-Ha-ras* and *c-myb* was not observed, particularly when one considers the fact that the *c-myb* gene, like the *c-myc* gene, in these cells is also amplified and overexpressed. The reasons for this apparent preferential affinity of pMC540 for the *c-myc* gene in L1210 cells remain unclear as of this writing. Nonetheless the importance of the c-myc protein in the DNA replication process has been clearly emphasized.[38,39] The association between activated *c-myc* gene (amplified or overexpressed) with cellular proliferation and cancer progression has also been reported.[36,40] Taken together, our data suggest that the *c-myc* gene might represent preferred targets for the Topo II-dependent antitumor agent pMC540. This behavior of pMC540 would be consistent with other antitumor drugs such as anthracyclines, epipodophyllotoxins and ellipticines, in view of their common mechanism of action with Topo II.

Clearly, a great deal of research work remains to be done to enhance our understanding of the relationships between pMC540 (as well as other novel compounds identified via the process of preactivation) induced damage within specific genomic regions, alterations in gene expression and preferential cytotoxicity towards certain types of tumor cells.

REFERENCES

1. Sager R. Tumor suppressor genes: The puzzle and the promise. Science 1989; 246:1406-10.
2. Watt R, Wang A, Schein P. Altered *c-myc* gene expression in Burkitt lymphoma cells following nitrogen mustard treatment. Proc Am Assoc Cancer Res 1986; 27:232.
3. Venturelli D, Lange B, Narni F et al. Prognostic significance of short term effect of chemotherapy on MYC and histone H3 m RNA levels in acute leukemia patients. Proc Natl Acad Sci USA 1988; 85:3590-4.
4. Greenberg M, Ziff E. Stimulation of 3T3 cells induces transcriptions of the c-fos proto-oncogene. Nature 1984; 311:433-38.
5. Kovacs E, Oppenheim J, and Young H. Induction of *c-fos* and *c-myc* expression in T-lymphocytes after treatment with recombinant interferon alpha. J Immunol 1986; 137:3649-51.
6. Kruiger W, Cooper J, Hunter T et al. Platelet-derived growth factor induces rapid but transient expression of the c-fos oncogene and protein. Nature 1984; 312:711-16.
7. Greenberg M, Ziff E, Greene L. Stimulation of neronal acetylcholine receptors induces rapid gene transcription. Science 1986; 234:80-3.
8. Morgan J, Cohen D, Hempstead J et al. Mapping patterns of *c-fos* expression in the central nervous system after seizure. Science 1987; 237:192-97.
9. Siebenblast U, Bressler P, Kelly K. Two distinct mechanisms of transcriptional control operate on *c-myc* during differentiation of HL-60 cells. Mol Cell Biol 1988; 8:867-74.
10. Trepel J, Colamonici O, Kelly K et al. Transcriptional inactivation of *c-myc* and the transferrin receptor in dibutyril cyclic-AMP-treated HL-60 cells. Mol Cell Biol 1987; 7:2644-48.
11. Reitsma P, Rothberg P, Astrin S et al. Rgulation of *c-myc* expression in HL-60 leukemic cells by a vitamin D metabolite. Nature 1983; 322:848-50.
12. Salomon DS, Perrotean J. Growth factors in cancer and their relationship to oncogenes. Cancer Invest 1986; 4:43-60.
13. Battey J, Moulding C, Taub R., Murphy W, Stewart T, Potter H, Lenoir G, Leder P. The human *c-myc* oncogene: structural conse-

quences of translocation into the IgH locus in Burkitt lymphoma. Cell 1983; 34:779-87.
14. Capon D, Chen E, Levinson A., Seeburg P, Goeddel D. Complete nucleotide sequences of the T24 human bladder carcinoma oncogene and its normal homologue. Nature (Lond.) 1983; 302:33-37.
15. Dalla Favera R, Wong-Staal, F, Gallo, R. Oncogene amplification in promyelocytic leukemia cell line HL-60 and primary leukemic cells of the same patient. Nature (Lond.) 1982; 299:61-63.
16. Schwab M, Ellison J, Busch M, Rosenau W, Varmus H, Bishop J. Enhanced expression of the human gene N-*myc* consequent to amplification of DNA may contribute to malignant progression of neuroblastoma. Proc Natl Acad Sci USA 1984; 81:4940–44.
17. Brodeur G, Seeger R, Schwab M, Varmus H, Bishop J. Amplification of N-*myc* in untreated human neuroblastomas correlates with advanced disease stage. Science (Wash. DC) 1984; 224:1121–24.
18. Watt R, Wang A, Schein P. Altered *c-myc* gene expression in Burkitt lymphoma cells following nitrogen mustard treatment. Proc Am Assoc Cancer Res 1986; 27:232.
19. Venturelli, D, Lange B, Narni F, Selleri L, Torelli U, Calabreta B. Prognostic significance of "short term" effects of chemotherapy on *MYC* and histone H3 mRNA levels in acute leukemia patients. Proc Natl Acad Sci USA, 1988; 85:3590-94.
20. Gulliya KS, Pervaiz S, Dowben RM, Matthews, JL. Tumor cell specific dark cytotoxicity of light-exposed merocyanine 540: implications for systemic therapy without light. Photochem Photobiol 1990; 51:831-38.
21. Chanh TC, Allan JS, Pervaiz S, Matthews JL, Gulliya KS. Preactivated merocyanine 540 inactivates HIV-1 and SIV: potential therapeutic and blood banking applications. J AIDS 1992; 5:188-95.
22. Wiggs, R. B., Lobprise, H.B., Matthews, J.L. and Gulliya, K.S. Effects of preactivated MC540 in the treatment of lymphocytic plasmacytic stomatitis in feline leukemia virus and feline immunodeficiecy virus positive cats. J. Veterinary Dentistry, 1993; 10:9-13.
23. Gulliya, K. S., Sharma, R. K., Matthews, J. L., Benniston, A. C., Harriman, A., and Nemunaitis, J. In vitro and in vivo growth suppression of MCF-7 human breast cancer by novel photoproducts and tamoxifen. Cancer 1994; 74:1725-32.
24. Sharma RK Gulliya KS. Growth inhibitory effects of pMC540 and merodantoin on established MCF-7 human breast tumor xenografts. In Vivo 1995; 9:103-108.
25. Lowry OH, Rosebrough N J, Farr AL, Randall RJ. Protein measurement with the folin ohenol reagent. J Biol Chem, 1951; 193:265-75.
26. Laemmle UK. Cleavage of structural proteins during the assembly of the head of bacteriophage T4. Nature 1970; 227:680-5.

27. Towbin H, Staehelin T, Gordon J. Electrophoretic transfer of proteins from polyacrylamide gels to nitrocellulose sheets: procedure and some applications. Proc Natl Acad Sci USA 1979; 76:4350-54.
28. Kaufmann S, Coffey D, Shaper J. Considerations in the isolation of rat liver nuclear matrix, nuclear envelope, and pore complex lamina. Exp Cell Res 1981; 132:105-23.
29. Persson H, Leder P. Nuclear localization and DNA binding properties of a protein expressed by human *c-myc* oncogene. Science, 1984; 225:718-21.
30. Futsher BW, Erickson LC. Changes in *c-myc* and *c-fos* expression in a human tumor cell line following exposure to bifunctional alkylating agents. Cancer Res 1990; 50: 62–66.
31. Gulliya KS, Frank B, Schneider U et al. Topoisomerase II-dependent novel antitumor compounds merocil and merodantoin induce apoptosis in Daudi cells. Anticancer Drugs 1994; 5:557-66.
32. Sharma RK, Arnold L, Gulliya KS. Correlation between DNA Topoisomerase II activity and cytotoxicity in pMC540 and merodantoin sensitive and resistant tumor breast cancer cells. Anticancer Research 1995; 15:295-304.
33. Osheroff N, Robinson MJ, Zechiedrich EL. Mechanism of the topoisimerase II-mediated DNA cleavage-religation reaction: Inhibition of DNA religation by antineoplastic drugs. In: Potmesil M Kohn KW, eds. DNA Topoisomerases in Cancer. Oxford University Press, 1991:230-39.
34. Rowe T, Kuffer G, Ross W. Inhibition of epipodophyllotoxin cytotoxicity by interference with topoisomerase-mediated DNA cleavage. Biochem Pharmacol 1985; 34:2483-87.
35. Riou JF, Multon E, Vilaren M-J et al. *In vivo* stimulation by antitumor drugs of the topoisomerase II induced cleavage sites in *c-myc* protooncogene. Biochem Biophys Res Commun 1986; 137:157-60.
36. Riou JF, Vilarem MJ, Larsen CJ et al. *In vivo* and *in vitro* stimulation by antitumor drugs of the topoisomerase II-induced cleavage sites of c-*myc* proto-oncogene. Natl Cancer Inst Monogr 1987; 4:41-47.
37. Dyson PJ, Rabbitts TH. Chromatin structure around the *c-myc* gene in Burkitt lymphomas with upstream and downstream translocation points. Proc Natl Acad Sci USA 1985; 82: 1984-88.
38. Studzinski GP, Brelvi ZS, Feldman SC et al. Participation of c-*myc* protein in DNA synthesis of human cells. Science 1986; 234:467-70.
39. Iguchi-Ariga SMM, Itani T, Kiji Y et al. Possible function of the c-*myc* product: promotion of cellular DNA replication. EMBO J 1987; 6:2365-71.
40. Little CD, Nau MM, Carney DN et al. Amplification and expression of the c-*myc* oncogene in human lung cancer cell lines. Nature 1983; 306:194-96.

EPILOGUE

Men with sore eyes....find the light painful, while darkness, which permits them to see nothing, is restful and agreeable.—Dio Chrysostom (40?-115?) Eleventh (Trojan) Discourse, II (tr. by J. W. Cohoon)

It is our wish that this book may become a contribution to the pedagogy of photobiology as well as new drug development. By way of concluding thoughts on preactivation, even at the risk of being redundant, I would like to summarize the salient points of this technology obtained to date. However, before proceeding with these points, I want to document a recollection of my first pleasant and uplifting experience that occurred soon after the discovery of preactivation during a site visit from NIH. After our presentation of the data on preactivation, Dr. Charles R. Smart, then Chief of Early Detection Branch at NCI, who, incidentally, was not a member of the site visit team, pulled me aside and said, "There are three things I want you to remember, 1) I consider this discovery a 'breakthrough' in the field; 2) it will not be easy but do not give up on it; and 3) the slides you have shown today, do not use them ever again because of their poor readability." In many ways Dr. Smart's comments have been a driving force for me. Needless to say, those slides, prepared in haste for the site visit, were promptly discarded and I have not yet given up on the discovery and development of preactivation technology. It is because of this discovery that a major limitation of photodynamic therapy, i.e. its dependence on light, has been eliminated for the first time in its over 90 years of documented history. The process of preactivation generates previously unknown chemotherapeutic agents that are not only effective against malignancies and viral infections but also easily tolerated. The mechanism of the formation of new agents is due to the reaction of singlet oxygen generated at excited states with the photoactive compound itself. As a result, the long held but completely unproven belief that singlet oxygen generated at excited states is the sole cause of cell kill, a cornerstone of photodynamic therapy, has been proven incorrect. It is interesting to note that while it is well established that singlet oxygen reacts indiscriminately with whatever happens to be around, the idea of its reaction with the compounds from which it is generated seems to annoy many in the field of photodynamic therapy. Even if I agree for a moment with the nay sayers, it is highly illogical that singlet oxygen would selectively spare the compound from which it was generated but react with everything else in sight. It is a physical impossibility given the nature of the beast. I think that proponents of this belief, perhaps for territorial reasons to keep photodynamic therapy apart from chemotherapy, have been successful only in keeping the photo chemotherapy from the main stream of clinical modalities. In fact, data presented here as well as data from numerous published reports indicate that at the molecular level the only difference between photo chemotherapy and chemotherapy is the use of chemical reaction-triggering photons. All subsequent reactions are very similar to most conventional chemotherapeutic agents such as adriamycin which is, for example, also known to produce in situ reactive oxygen species. Even though "...history is replete with accounts of discoveries usually met with rebuff and denial"* , all is not lost because many visionary scientists have already confirmed that pre-illumination or preactivation of photoactive compounds leads to the generation of new photoproducts, as described in chapter 2.

Nonetheless, the discovery of preactivation has also been instrumental in illustrating that drugs that destroy more than one type of cancer and spare the host should not be considered useless as dictated by the National Cancer Institute's current criteria of drug selection for further research and development. Thus, in accordance with the central goal of cancer therapy, the first criterion for drug selection should be re-written to read that the new agent must be cytotoxic to one or more types of tumor cells and it must

**Thomas A Kuhn, The Structure of Scientific Revolutions, 2nd ed., Chicago, University of Chicago Press, 1970.*

be highly sparing of the normal cells and tissues, i.e. the host, period.

The commonly held belief that an antitumor agent cannot be an antiviral agent as well is also incorrect. Data presented in this book clearly demonstrate that preactivated compounds are effective antitumor and antiviral agents. This dual action of certain compounds is certainly not a novelty, e.g. many photoactive compounds are also known to possess both antitumor and antiviral properties. How an agent can destroy two distinctly different targets such as a tumor cell and virus is the question that probably forms the basis of the erroneously held belief mentioned above. However, if one were to take a closer look at these two targets, it would be abundantly clear that while differences between the two are obvious, similarities do exist. For example, it is well-established from the published literature that there are many similarities between the viral envelope and the plasma membrane of the host cell from which the virion originates. These similarities offer a window through which cytotoxic as well as virucidal effects could be mediated by certain compounds. Preactivated chemotherapeutic agents appear to exploit these similarities between tumor cells and enveloped viruses. This view is further supported by the fact that these preactivated agents were found to be totally ineffective against non-enveloped viruses. Thus, blanket statements or customary beliefs, that an antitumor agent cannot function as an antiviral agent or vice versa, are based on entirely unscientific grounds and serve only to prevent the development of highly beneficial agents for the treatment of malignancies and viral infections. Needless to say, this area of research remains open for further exploitation, pending rejection of existing paradigms.

Thus, systematic experiments performed over the last nine years have clearly demonstrated the feasibility of the novel approach of preactivation as well as the resultant new chemotherapeutic agents in vitro and in vivo models. Having done so, one must ask, is it ethical to deny terminal patients, such as those with terminal stages of prostate or breast cancer or those infected with HIV, an opportunity to choose an uncertain treatment which may well be beneficial by not making agents such as pMC540 available to them? When such an opportunity is denied by someone other than the patient, can it really be called an act of human rights? Whose rights are we talking about here, the regulatory agencies or the patients? Why are terminal patients not allowed to try anything they desire? Are we afraid that some injury more serious than death may be inflicted by the treatment, or are we truly afraid of losing control over patients in the name of protection? It is obvious that if those responsible for denying such an opportunity were to become afflicted with a terminal disease themselves, they would scour the world to find a cure. Making someone else's life less valuable than one's own is most certainly unethical. People should not be forced to sacrifice their lives until another drug is approved. It is simply not ethical! The Hippocratic maxim *primo non nocere* which means 'above all things do no harm' is certainly applicable when preventing someone from choosing causes ultimate harm.

It does not have to be this way. While the value of regulations for nonterminal diseases is well recognized, for terminal patients there is a lot of room between "either FDA approved drugs or no treatment at all." For terminal patients, guidelines could be established such that promising experimental drugs become easily accessible without exploitation of these patients. For example, experimental agents could be approved for a very limited number (e.g. 6) of patients if the following simple conditions are met:

1.) The drug is relatively safe as demonstrated even by the very preliminary data in one or more animal models.
2.) The cost of the drug will be absorbed by the provider in exchange of data.
3.) Informed consent of the patient with full disclosure of the existing information about the experimental drug.
4.) The drug will be given under the supervision of a physician.
5.) Further approval of additional patients will be strictly dependent upon the absence of severe toxicity, and some evidence of benefit to the patients over a reasonable period of time say three to six months.

Naturally, these guidelines are provided as an example and should be modified or added to in accordance with the individual situation, as long as the rule of common sense and patients' well-being is kept as the central goal. Some evidence of this kind of appropriate action is already visible in the approval of bone marrow transplantation from a baboon to one HIV infected patient. This kind of limited approval at an accelerated pace is what's needed and it certainly is worthy of applause that someone is listening.

In conclusion, there is only praise in changing the drum beat to be in tune with the growing knowledge and awareness of truth. It is our sincere hope that at least this time the following quotation is proven wrong.

"A new scientific truth does not triumph by convincing its opponents and making them see the light, but rather because its opponents eventually die and a new generation grows up that is familiar with it." —Max Planck, 1949.

INDEX

Page numbers in italics denote figures (f) or tables (t).

V

W

Z

GPSR Compliance

The European Union's (EU) General Product Safety Regulation (GPSR) is a set of rules that requires consumer products to be safe and our obligations to ensure this.

If you have any concerns about our products, you can contact us on ProductSafety@springernature.com

In case Publisher is established outside the EU, the EU authorized representative is:

Springer Nature Customer Service Center GmbH
Europaplatz 3
69115 Heidelberg, Germany

Batch number: 10615115

Printed by Printforce, the Netherlands